Prediabetes

2nd Edition

by Simon Poole, MD and Amy Riolo

Authors of *Diabetes For Dummies* and
Diabetes Cookbook For Dummies
Alan L. Rubin, MD

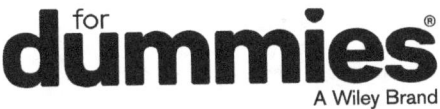

A Wiley Brand

Prediabetes For Dummies®, 2nd Edition

Published by: **John Wiley & Sons, Inc.**, 111 River Street, Hoboken, NJ 07030-5774, www.wiley.com

For general information on our other products and services, please contact our Customer Care Department within the U.S. at 877-762-2974, outside the U.S. at 317-572-3993, or fax 317-572-4002. For technical support, please visit https://hub.wiley.com/community/support/dummies.

Wiley publishes in a variety of print and electronic formats and by print-on-demand. Some material included with standard print versions of this book may not be included in e-books or in print-on-demand. If this book refers to media such as a CD or DVD that is not included in the version you purchased, you may download this material at http://booksupport.wiley.com. For more information about Wiley products, visit www.wiley.com.

Library of Congress Control Number is available from the publisher.

ISBN 978-1-394-36116-8 (pbk); ISBN 978-1-394-36117-5 (ebk); ISBN 978-1-394-36118-2 (epdf)

Printed and bound by CPI Group (UK) Ltd, Croydon, CR0 4YY

C9781394361168_160226

The manufacturer's authorized representative according to the EU General Product Safety Regulation is Wiley-VCH GmbH, Boschstr. 12, 69469 Weinheim, Germany, e-mail: Product_Safety@wiley.com.

Contents at a Glance

Table of Contents

Introduction

Prediabetes is a medical condition that is rapidly on the rise. It's expected that over 470 million people will have prediabetes globally in the next five years. It is estimated that 80% of the people who have prediabetes don't even realize that they have it. Because prediabetes can lead to serious health complications such as the onset of heart disease, diabetes, and stroke, learning how to prevent and reverse it is important. While prediabetes should be taken seriously, a diagnosis doesn't mean that it's time to panic. By maintaining a calm, practical, and even enjoyable approach to healthful eating and lifestyle strategies, you and those you love can prevent the onset of diabetes while enjoying yourself in the process.

Why Do We Need This Book?

The growing epidemic of prediabetes and diabetes call for accurate, concise, and helpful information that will help to disrupt the current negative trends. By providing those with prediabetes the information they need to take charge of their health and prevent the onset of diabetes itself, this book can help you and your loved ones to live their best lives.

Having a prediabetes diagnosis means that your blood sugar levels are higher than normal, but they are not high enough to be in the diabetes category. While you may not see drastic warning signs with prediabetes, a doctor's diagnosis is your warning sign to make the positive changes which will keep you healthy.

We define prediabetes clearly in Chapter 1. Prediabetes is not usually associated with all the bad complications of diabetes, which we discuss in Chapter 3, but it alone may be associated with some heart problems. And prediabetes is not only the stage before diabetes. It may also be the stage before high blood pressure (*prehypertension*) or high cholesterol. All the abnormalities that lead to prediabetes (that can go on to diabetes) are also to blame for the development of prehypertension (that can go on to high blood pressure) and mildly elevated cholesterol (that can go on to hypercholesterolemia). By helping you to reverse prediabetes, we're also helping you to reverse the other two conditions. So, you are basically getting three books for the price of one. What a deal!

Approaching this book with the knowledge that you *can* reverse prediabetes is important. If there is one point that we want to make clear, it's that you are not doomed to develop diabetes just because you have prediabetes. You can still enjoy optimal health and using this book as a guide enables you to do so. If you reverse prediabetes, you will probably reverse prehypertension and mildly elevated cholesterol as well. Chapters 8 through 21 provide everything you need to know to do this.

About This Book

This book is an excellent resource for what you need to know about prediabetes — and a lot about diabetes as well. (You can find everything you need to know about diabetes in an excellent book called *Diabetes For Dummies,* the 6th edition of which we wrote a few years ago.)

You don't have to read this book from start to finish (but it wouldn't hurt). You can pick up the book and start reading anywhere you want. If you want to know what prediabetes is, start with Chapter 1. If you want to know what factors lead to prediabetes, Part 1 provides the answers. Getting a diagnosis is taken up in Part 2, while Part 3 discusses creating a healthy lifestyle. Part 4 teaches you the ways that the Mediterranean diet can work for you. Part 5 tells you how to avoid or reverse prediabetes.

Our aim, with this book, is to empower you to embrace science-based approaches to creating a healthy lifestyle. Developing a healthy relationship with food, achieving and maintaining a healthy weight, living an active lifestyle, and managing stress and seeking joy, are important factors which we illustrate throughout this guide to help prevent you from developing diabetes.

Conventions Used in This Book

The sugar in your blood is called *glucose,* and too-high glucose leads to many of the complications of diabetes. But the white sugar you eat is not glucose; it's sucrose. And many other sugars exist, such as fructose, maltose, and galactose. So we don't use just the word *sugar* in this book; we call the particular sugar by its proper name.

When we mention a level of blood sugar (glucose), it is shown in units called *milligrams per deciliter* (mg/dL). I don't mean to confuse you, but the rest of the world uses the International System of units called, in this case, *millimoles per liter* (mmol/L). You can convert mg/dL to mmol/L as you cross the border of the United States into Canada simply by dividing the mg/dL by 18. For example, a blood glucose of 100 mg/dL is 5.5 mmol/L.

Two major types of diabetes exist: *Type 1* diabetes mellitus and *Type 2* diabetes mellitus. We refer to them as *Type 1* and *Type 2* diabetes in this book.

We discuss nutrition, exercise, and lifestyle frequently in this book because of how they affect your overall health, which in turn affects your susceptibility to prediabetes and diabetes.

Finally, in Chapter 15, Chef Amy Riolo (one of the authors) includes more than 25 complete meal recipes to try. Each of these recipes is packed not only with flavor, but with balanced micronutrients and powerful plant compounds which can reduce inflammation and help balance blood sugar. If you're a vegetarian, look for the tomato next to the recipe name that indicates the recipe does not contain meat, poultry, or fish.

What You Don't Have to Read

Everyone is different. You may have received a thorough explanation of what prediabetes is from your doctor already, and you're just here to discover how to manage it. In that case, you can skip to Part 3. If you're unfamiliar with what prediabetes is, how to help a loved one, how to prevent children from being diagnosed, and so forth, however, reading Part 4 in its entirety is a good idea. The Part of Tens section offers four chapters that are full of concise, helpful information that are great to reference from time to time on your wellness journey.

Foolish Assumptions

We assume that your mind is a blank when it comes to the actual scientific differences between prediabetes and diabetes. Therefore, you won't suddenly come up against a term that you have never seen before without finding an immediate definition of that term. On the other hand, if you already know something about the subject, you can expect to find much greater detail. Throughout the book, the most important points are clearly marked using tools such as icons (which we explain in a moment).

We also assume that you'd like to know as much as possible, and as many ways as possible in which you can help yourself or others reverse diabetes. For this reason, we explain each of the tips and strategies that are available currently to help you do so.

How This Book Is Organized

This book has six parts, and you don't have to start at Part 1. Each part is self-contained. In fact, each chapter is self-contained, so if you see a chapter title that really excites you such as "Cooking and Eating for Health and Enjoyment," feel free to jump right in there. Here is a brief synopsis of what you can find in each part of this book.

Part 1: Confronting the Prediabetes Epidemic

This introductory part gives you a foundation of understanding as to what prediabetes is all about. Dr. Simon Poole starts with a discussion of how prediabetes originates. From there, he moves on to talk about when you should suspect that you have developed prediabetes. What are the elements of your family history, your personal history, and your current lifestyle that suggest this diagnosis? Moving right along, he traces the factors that convert prediabetes to diabetes. Then he offers a general discussion about stopping this conversion before it happens.

Part 2: Getting a Diagnosis

The second part of the book defines the Metabolic Syndrome and how to spot it. It also teaches how essential tests are performed and how to interpret results. In this part, Dr. Simon Poole also discusses special conditions including children, the elderly, and other life stages in which prediabetes is prevalent. Getting the proper diagnosis is the first step to transforming your health.

Part 3: Food and Other Factors: Creating a Healthy Lifestyle

What you discover in these chapters should make it clear to you that prediabetes, as well as Type 2 diabetes, is promoted by unhealthy lifestyle habits, which means both conditions can be reversed by adopting healthier lifestyle habits.

The first lifestyle habit to consider is the food you eat. Next, you want to deal with your weight by maintaining an active lifestyle. Exercise is an important component of a healthy lifestyle, which can help you burn calories and gain muscle. Finally, taking steps toward minimizing stress can help you manage prediabetes successfully.

Part 4: The Benefits of the Mediterranean Diet

Untreated or poorly managed diabetes can cause low blood glucose (*hypoglycemia*) and very high blood glucose (*hyperglycemia*). These conditions have a very definite effect on your quality of life and need to be prevented.

Next are the long-term complications that take ten or more years of diabetes to develop but can be devastating. Blindness, kidney failure, nerve disease, and heart disease are the factors to fear in this regard. But you are never going to have any of these complications because you are going to reverse your prediabetes, so it never gets to diabetes!

A special category of long-term complications are sexual complications and the complications of pregnancy. These situations warrant their own chapter. (It's not X-rated, so feel free to read it even when the kids are around.)

The Mediterranean diet has been selected as the best overall diet in the world and one of its strengths is being efficient in helping those who follow it reverse and prevent diabetes. This section teaches how to make the Mediterranean diet work for you. From adapting a healthful approach towards food to discovering which types of foods are best for diabetes, this part enables you to power-charge your meal plan with ingredients that have stood the test of time and continue to help people live better and longer.

Part 5: Avoiding or Reversing Prediabetes

Now it's time to head to the kitchen! Creating homemade meals, no matter how simple, for yourself or others is one of the best ways to take charge of your diet. In Chapter 15, we cook together and enjoy the healthful and delicious food we make. You unearth delicious and nutritious recipes to enjoy at breakfast snack-time, lunch, dinner, and for dessert. In this chapter, Chef and coauthor Amy Riolo provides you with recipes that feature nutritious yet inexpensive ingredients in a variety of ways that can be enjoyed by a wide range of palettes.

Can medications help to reverse prediabetes? You find out in Chapter 16, and you also find out whether any vitamins or supplements may make a difference.

To put all your new knowledge together, we created Chapter 17, which features a complete plan for a three-month health makeover. Sometimes you need structure in order to succeed. This chapter tells you what to eat, what exercise to do, and everything else you need to know to create the healthy habits which can help you for life.

Part 6: The Part of Tens

No *For Dummies* book is complete without this part. You can read ten myths about prediabetes, ten staples to keep in your kitchen, ten ways to stop prediabetes in its tracks, and ten ways to help kids prevent and reverse diabetes.

Icons Used in This Book

The icons alert you to information you must know, information you should know, and information you may find interesting but can live without.

REMEMBER

When you see this icon, it means the information is essential and you should be aware of it.

TECHNICAL STUFF

This icon informs you of information that may be useful but not extremely important.

TIP

This icon marks important information that can save you time and energy.

WARNING

This icon alerts you to important information that can assist you with managing prediabetes.

Beyond the Book

In addition to the abundance of information and guidance related to prediabetes that we provide in this book, you get access to even more help and information online at *Dummies.com*. Check out this book's online Cheat Sheet. Just go to *www.dummies.com* and search for "Prediabetes For Dummies Cheat Sheet."

1

Confronting the Prediabetes Epidemic

Chapter **1**

The Origins and Dangers of Prediabetes

Prediabetes is a condition in which blood sugar (in the form of glucose) levels are higher than normal but not yet high enough to be diagnosed as Type 2 diabetes. It signals that the body is starting to have trouble managing blood glucose effectively.

While prediabetes itself may not cause noticeable symptoms, high blood glucose increases the risk of developing Type 2 diabetes, heart disease, and other medical problems if left unaddressed. Even if blood glucose levels don't rise progressively to a diagnosis of Type 2 diabetes, having higher than normal average blood glucose levels does increase the risk of some of the same health complications that are associated with Type 2 diabetes including heart disease and strokes, kidney and eyes diseases as well as in increased risk of neurological problems including dementia.

REMEMBER

Although the prefix "pre" may suggest that prediabetes inevitably leads to diabetes, this is certainly not the case and there are many people who would not be predestined to develop Type 2 diabetes.

Diagnosing prediabetes is crucial because it may be the critical step before developing diabetes. As you find out in this book, diabetes is associated with complications that may cause considerable physical and mental discomfort at best and be life-threatening at worst. So you don't want to go there.

Even if you go on to develop diabetes, all is not lost. You can use the suggestions found here to avoid further complications. You can't get rid of the diagnosis, but you can get rid of the problems.

In this chapter, you discover how to differentiate among three physical states: normal health, prediabetes, and diabetes. We explain that prediabetes is a recent phenomenon, which parallels the epidemic of obesity and lack of exercise in countries around the world.

Next, you discover who is affected by prediabetes and which groups of people are at the highest risk. We also touch on special considerations for children and the elderly at risk for prediabetes.

Finally, we focus on the costs of prediabetes, which are not only monetary. We explain that even though prediabetes is often considered a benign condition and not a disease, changes occur in the body of a person with prediabetes that may not be benign after all.

Recognizing a Global Problem

Prediabetes is increasingly recognized as a major public health concern in the United States, Europe, and around the world. What makes prediabetes particularly worrying is its silent nature and a vast majority of those who have it are unaware. In the United States, for example, the Centers for Disease Control and Prevention (CDC) estimates that about 96 million adults, or nearly 38 percent of the adult population, have prediabetes. Yet over 80 percent of these people don't know they're affected. The situation is similarly concerning in Europe. According to the International Diabetes Federation, over 36 million people in Europe are thought to have prediabetes. In the UK, National Health Service figures suggest that around 5 million people may be living with prediabetes, sometimes referred to as "non-diabetic hyperglycemia."

Globally, the International Diabetes Federation estimates that more than 540 million adults may be affected by prediabetes. While high-income countries still bear much of the burden, the problem is accelerating in low- and middle-income nations due to rapid urbanization, changes in diet, and increasingly sedentary lifestyles. What is especially concerning is the strong association between prediabetes and the eventual development of Type 2 diabetes. Without intervention, as many as 70 percent of people with prediabetes will go on to develop diabetes, often within five to ten years.

Taking control of prediabetes

The good news is that prediabetes is being identified more frequently with increased screening and can often be reversed or managed through the lifestyle changes described throughout this book. In this chapter, you discover some of the basics about prediabetes and its impact on health.

Here are some encouraging facts about managing prediabetes:

>> Without intervention, about 15–30 percent of people with prediabetes will develop Type 2 diabetes within five years. This means that while a substantial proportion do progress, it is not inevitable. Many do not develop diabetes, especially with lifestyle changes.

>> Up to 50 percent of Type 2 diabetes cases can be prevented or delayed with appropriate lifestyle modifications, such as weight loss, healthy eating, and increased physical activity.

>> A substantial number of people with prediabetes can reverse the condition through lifestyle changes such as losing a modest amount of weight, eating more healthfully, and becoming more physically active.

>> With the right changes, many people are able to bring their blood glucose levels back into the normal range, often avoiding the progression to Type 2 diabetes altogether.

>> Even if blood glucose doesn't return fully to normal, lifestyle improvements can still make a big difference — slowing or stopping the progression to diabetes and lowering the risk of serious complications.

>> While not everyone may fully reverse prediabetes, the majority of people who make and sustain these changes can significantly improve how their body handles glucose and reduce their long-term health risks.

Embodying the Spectrum

Every cell in the human body needs energy to function, and one of the body's primary sources of this energy is *glucose* — a simple sugar derived from the food we eat. When we consume carbohydrates such as bread, fruit, rice, or pasta, our digestive system breaks them down into glucose, which is then absorbed into the bloodstream. Protein and fat can also be converted into glucose by the body, particularly when carbohydrate intake is low. This blood glucose is then transported around the body and taken up by cells, where it's either used immediately for energy or stored for later use.

To ensure that blood glucose levels remain within a healthy range, our bodies rely on a carefully balanced system of regulation. A key player in this process is the hormone insulin, which is produced by the pancreas. When glucose enters the bloodstream after a meal, insulin is released to help move the glucose from the blood into the cells. This keeps blood glucose levels from rising too high. Between meals or during periods of physical activity, the body taps into its glucose stores to keep energy levels stable.

However, this finely tuned system can be disrupted by various aspects of lifestyle. Dietary habits, portion sizes, levels of physical activity, the presence of excess body fat, and the quality of sleep can all influence how efficiently the body regulates blood glucose. Genetic factors also play an important role. When the balance tips, either because the body doesn't respond properly to insulin or because insulin production declines, glucose can start to build up in the bloodstream. Over time, chronically elevated blood glucose levels can damage blood vessels and organs, contributing to serious complications such as heart disease, kidney problems, and vision loss.

This risk doesn't appear overnight; it increases gradually. There is a spectrum of blood glucose regulation that ranges from healthy and optimal, through intermediate stages where glucose levels are mildly elevated in prediabetes, to persistently high levels that meet the criteria for diabetes. Everyone, whether they are aware of it or not, is somewhere on this spectrum. Some people manage their blood glucose levels very efficiently, while others may struggle due to lifestyle factors, genetics, or a combination of both.

Understanding where you fall on this spectrum is important, and fortunately there are reliable ways to measure how well your body is handling glucose over time. These measurements — such as fasting glucose, HbA1c, or glucose tolerance tests — are explored in more detail later in this chapter. For now, it's worth remembering that blood glucose regulation is something that affects everyone, and that the way each of us live our daily lives has a powerful influence on how well our bodies manage this essential energy source.

Going from normal to prediabetes

The diagnosis of prediabetes is made the same way that a diagnosis of diabetes is made: by doing a blood glucose test in the laboratory.

Many countries, including the United States, report blood glucose levels in milligrams per deciliter (mg/dL), while many other regions such as Europe and the UK use millimoles per liter (mmol/L). Both units measure the same thing, but the values differ due to the conversion factor between the two systems.

The critical *values* (numbers) in the test results are as follows:

- A normal fasting blood glucose result is less than 100 mg/dL (5.6 mmol/L).

- Prediabetes is diagnosed when the fasting blood glucose is between 100 and 125 mg/dL (5.6–6.9 mmol/L) on more than one occasion.

- Diabetes is diagnosed when the fasting blood glucose is 126 mg/dL (7 mmol/L) or greater on more than one occasion.

- A normal blood glucose level two hours after eating 75 grams of glucose is less than 140 mg/dL (7.8 mmol/L).

- Prediabetes is diagnosed when the glucose two hours after eating 75 grams of glucose is between 140 and 199 mg/dL (7.8–11.1 mmol/L) on more than one occasion.

- Diabetes is diagnosed when the glucose two hours after eating 75 grams of glucose is 200 mg/dL (11.1 mmol/L) or greater on more than one occasion.

Table 1-1 is a summary of these values using mg/dL units.

TABLE 1-1　　　**Normal, Prediabetic, and Diabetic Glucose Values**

Type of Test	Normal	Prediabetes	Diabetes
Fasting blood glucose	Less than 100 mg/dL	100–125 mg/dL	126 mg/dL or greater
Blood glucose two hours after eating 75 grams of glucose	Less than 140 mg/dL	140–199 mg/dL	200 mg/dL or greater

In recent years, another laboratory test called HbA1c has become a widely used way of diagnosing and monitoring both prediabetes and diabetes. HbA1c stands for glycated hemoglobin, which refers to the percentage of red blood cells that have glucose attached to them. Because red blood cells live for, and are replaced in, a cycle of around three months, this test reflects a person's average blood glucose level over the previous two to three months — rather than just at the moment of testing, such as a fasting glucose or glucose tolerance test does.

The use of HbA1c in diagnosing diabetes became more common after it was endorsed by major organizations such as the American Diabetes Association (ADA) and the World Health Organization (WHO) around 2009–2011. One of the main reasons for its popularity is practicality. Unlike glucose tests, HbA1c doesn't require fasting, and it isn't affected by short-term factors such as recent meals, stress, or illness. That makes it more convenient for both patients and healthcare providers.

According to current guidelines:

>> An HbA1c below 5.7 percent (which is below 39 mmol/mol) is considered normal.

>> A level between 5.7 percent and 6.4 percent (39–47 mmol/mol) indicates prediabetes.

>> A level of 6.5 percent or higher (48 mmol/mol or above), confirmed by a repeat test, signals diabetes.

While HbA1c is now frequently used to diagnose prediabetes because of its reliability and convenience, with a single blood test without the need for fasting, it is also useful for monitoring how well prediabetes is managed over time. However, it's worth noting that HbA1c results can be less reliable in certain individuals, for example, those with anemia, certain blood disorders, or recent blood loss, so healthcare professionals may choose alternative tests when needed.

REMEMBER

These definitions are arbitrary. They have changed in the past, and they may do so again depending on scientific studies. For example, a fasting glucose result of greater than 140 mg/dL (7.8 mmol/L) used to be the cutoff point for a diagnosis of diabetes. Then doctors discovered that people who had fasting glucose levels below 140 mg/dL suffered from the complications of diabetes without having a diagnosis of diabetes. So, they lowered the level for the diagnosis to 126 mg/dL (7 mmol/L). Unfortunately, even some people with fasting blood glucose levels below 126 have shown up with complications of diabetes.

You should be familiar with some other terms for these levels of blood glucose, because you likely can read or hear about them:

>> *Impaired fasting glucose* (IFG) is another name for the condition where the fasting blood glucose is between 100 and 125 mg/dL (5.6–6.9 mmol/L) after an overnight fast.

>> *Impaired glucose tolerance* (IGT) is another name for the condition where the blood glucose is between 140 and 199 mg/dL (7.8–11.1 mmol/L) two hours after eating 75 grams of glucose.

Some people have impaired fasting glucose, while others have impaired glucose tolerance. Still others have both conditions combined, so the total number of people with prediabetes is *not* the sum of the people with IFG plus the people with IGT.

Other terms that you may hear should be disregarded because they have no clear meaning and are no longer used scientifically. These include:

>> Borderline diabetes

>> Touch of sugar

Understanding diabetes

Two major types of diabetes are called *Type 1 diabetes mellitus* (T1DM) and *Type 2 diabetes mellitus* (T2DM). (If you want to find out exactly what distinguishes them, pick up our book *Diabetes For Dummies*, which is also published by Wiley.) Here's a grossly oversimplified overview:

>> Type 1 is an autoimmune disease that usually occurs in children.

>> Type 2 may occur in either children or adults and is often associated with risk factors such as being overweight and having high blood pressure.

When diabetes develops in Type 2, the body still has plenty of insulin but not enough to keep the blood glucose in the normal range because the body resists the action of insulin.

The word *prediabetes* in this book refers to the period between normal blood glucose control and Type 2 diabetes.

Knowing the Recent History of Prediabetes

In this section, we discuss the reason for the development of the term *prediabetes*, as well as the fact that prediabetes is not an entirely benign condition.

Needing new language

The term *prediabetes* hasn't been around long. In fact, it was first used in 2002. It was introduced by the American Diabetes Association (ADA) and by Tommy G. Thompson, the health and human services secretary at the time.

A number of reasons for the introduction of this term were:

>> The terms *impaired fasting glucose* and *impaired glucose tolerance* were meaningless to patients and required a lot of explaining.

>> Other terms, such as *touch of sugar* and *borderline diabetes,* were generally meaningless.

>> Studies such as the Diabetes Prevention Program showed that diet and exercise resulting in a weight loss as little as 5 to 7 percent of someone's initial weight would lower the incidence of Type 2 diabetes by up to 58 percent.

>> A broadly understandable term was needed so that patients could know where they were and where they had to go with respect to diabetes. These people stood to benefit from lifestyle modification and other treatments.

Studies at the time showed that most people with prediabetes would go on to develop diabetes within ten years unless they made relatively modest changes in diet and exercise. Therefore, the ADA and Thompson put together an expert panel of doctors and other diabetes experts. The panel report stated that intervention in prediabetes is critical for three reasons:

>> Just having glucose levels in the prediabetic range puts a person at a 50 percent greater risk of a heart attack or stroke.

>> The development of Type 2 diabetes can be delayed or prevented by modest lifestyle change.

>> For many people, modest changes in lifestyle can turn back the clock and return elevated blood glucose levels to normal.

Along with the new term, the ADA recommended that physicians begin to screen their patients for prediabetes at age 45. Screening was especially important for people who answered yes to these questions:

>> Do you have a relative with Type 2 diabetes or heart disease?

>> Are you overweight or obese?

>> Do you have high blood pressure?

>> Do you have a sedentary lifestyle?

>> Do you have high levels of triglycerides and/or low levels of HDL cholesterol (both being types of fats measured in a blood test)?

> **»** Do you belong to a higher-risk ethnic group, such as African American, Latino, or Asian American/Pacific Islander?

> **»** Do you have apple-shaped rather than pear-shaped weight distribution? This means your excess weight is around your stomach rather than your hips.

> **»** For women who have had children, did you develop diabetes during the pregnancy or have a baby who weighed more than 9 pounds at birth?

> **»** For women, is there a history of *polycystic ovarian syndrome,* a condition that may include lack of periods, infertility, and increased hair on the body?

Understanding the Risks

Prediabetes may not be associated with all the problems of diabetes, but your body may be developing some reversible damage if you have this condition. We discuss the most important issues here.

Heart attacks and strokes

People with blood sugar levels above the healthy range in the prediabetes zone face a significantly increased risk of heart disease and stroke. Research shows the relative risk of these cardiovascular events can be up to twice as high compared to those with consistently healthy blood sugar. If blood sugar rises further into the diabetes range, the risk increases even more. These relationships are strongly supported by large, long-term studies, though it is important to note that other factors such as blood pressure, cholesterol, and lifestyle habits also play a role.

Eye health: Retinopathy

Damage to the small blood vessels in the eye, known as *retinopathy*, is a well-known complication of diabetes, but it can also occur when blood sugar is only moderately elevated. Studies have shown that the risk of developing eye problems rises steadily as glucose levels increase, even before reaching the diabetes threshold. There is no clear cut-off below which risk disappears, but the closer blood sugar is to the normal range, the lower the risk of vision-related complications.

Brain health and dementia

Higher blood sugar levels are associated with an increased risk of cognitive decline and dementia, including Alzheimer's disease. Research indicates that individuals with elevated blood glucose in the prediabetes range tend to perform worse on memory and thinking tests than those with lower, healthier glucose levels. The risk of developing Alzheimer's disease is about twice as high for people with diabetes, and those with prediabetes also show measurable declines in brain function. While these findings show strong associations, it is not yet clear if high blood sugar directly causes dementia or if shared risk factors are involved.

Quality of life and daily function

Living with prediabetes can impact daily life. Studies have found that people with elevated glucose levels report lower quality of life, including more fatigue, reduced work productivity, and increased absenteeism. On average, individuals in this group lose several weeks of productive time each year compared to those with healthy blood sugar.

Chronic kidney disease

Growing evidence shows that people with moderately elevated blood sugar have a higher risk of developing chronic kidney disease (CKD). A large meta-analysis found that those with higher-than-normal glucose had about a 12 percent increased risk of CKD compared to those with normal blood sugar, after accounting for other risk factors. Recent studies have found that the prevalence of CKD in this group can be as high as 16.5 percent, compared to 15.3 percent in the general population and nearly 30 percent in those with diabetes. Other research has shown that more than one third of people with elevated glucose show early signs of kidney damage, such as protein in the urine or reduced kidney function. While these studies demonstrate a clear association, it is not yet certain that higher blood sugar directly causes kidney disease, as other factors such as high blood pressure and cholesterol often coexist.

Overall mortality

Elevated blood sugar, even if not in the diabetes range, has been linked to a higher risk of premature death from all causes. Large population studies find that people with higher-than-normal glucose have an increased risk of dying from heart disease, stroke, kidney failure, and some cancers compared to those with normal blood sugar. While these associations are consistent, it is important to recognize that other lifestyle factors, such as obesity, smoking, and lack of physical activity, may also contribute to the increased risk.

Risk of cancer

Recent research suggests that people with moderately elevated blood sugar may have a higher risk of developing certain cancers, including pancreatic, liver, endometrial, stomach, colorectal, breast, and gallbladder cancers. For example, a 2024 meta-analysis found a 42 percent higher risk of pancreatic cancer among people with elevated glucose compared to those with normal levels. However, the relationship between blood sugar and cancer is complex and may be influenced by other factors such as excess weight, poor diet, and physical inactivity, which often accompany higher glucose levels. Therefore, while there is a clear association, it is not certain that elevated blood sugar directly causes cancer.

REMEMBER

Even though prediabetes is not as serious as diabetes, it does involve medical deterioration. The longer you allow yourself to have prediabetes, the greater the damage. Start to reverse it now!

Realizing Who Is Affected

Some groups of people are affected by prediabetes more than others, and they may even be affected when their blood glucose levels are lower than the levels that currently define prediabetes. (In the earlier section "Going from normal to prediabetes," We spell out those levels.)

Prediabetes rates of about 38 percent in the adult US population are now considered similar across major racial and ethnic groups when age-adjusted. While earlier studies suggested some differences, current research shows that non-Hispanic White, non-Hispanic Black, Hispanic or Latino, Asian American, and American Indian and Alaska Native adults all experience prediabetes at comparable rates. This means that elevated blood sugar before the onset of diabetes is a shared challenge for many Americans, regardless of background.

However, disparities remain in the progression from prediabetes to diabetes. Adults from non-Hispanic Black, Hispanic or Latino, Asian American, and American Indian and Alaska Native backgrounds are more likely to develop diabetes compared to non-Hispanic White adults. For example, the CDC reports that the age-adjusted prevalence of diagnosed diabetes is 12.1 percent in non-Hispanic Black adults, 11.7 percent in Hispanic or Latino adults, 13.6 percent in American Indian and Alaska Native adults, and 9.1 percent in non-Hispanic Asian adults, compared to 6.9 percent in non-Hispanic White adults. These differences are influenced by a variety of factors, including genetics, access to healthcare, socioeconomic status, and the impact of social determinants of health.

Approaching these statistics with respect and sensitivity is important. Differences in health outcomes among racial and ethnic groups are shaped by a complex mix of factors, including historical and ongoing inequities in healthcare access, neighborhood resources, and opportunities for healthy living.

WARNING

These numbers reflect patterns seen in large populations and should never be used to make assumptions about individuals or communities. Addressing these disparities and inequalities is a moral imperative and requires culturally sensitive prevention and care, as well as efforts to improve access to healthy food, safe places to be active, and high-quality health care for everyone.

Ensuring that proper education on healthful diets, lifestyle, and the strategies for being able to implement them is available to all communities (especially those which are underserved) is integral to transform the historical patterns that evidence suggests. Whether it's teaching nutrition classes, offering educational programming on fitness, cooking classes, or giving people tips to fit the lifestyle habits into their daily life with ease, every amount of time and money spent on education offers enormous benefit.

Considering children and adolescents

By 2023, the Centers for Disease Control and Prevention (CDC) estimated that 8.4 million US adolescents aged 12 to 17, about 32.7 percent, have prediabetes, a dramatic increase from earlier years. This rise in prediabetes among young people is closely linked to the ongoing epidemic of childhood obesity which is closely associated with the development of prediabetes.

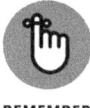

REMEMBER

The prevalence of obesity among children ages 6 to 11 in the United States has remained a serious concern. According to the CDC, as of 2017–2020, approximately 20.7 percent of children ages 6 to 11 were classified as having obesity. Among adolescents aged 12 to 19, the rate was even higher, with 22.2 percent affected by obesity. These figures reflect a continued rise from previous decades and underscore how high rates of childhood and adolescent obesity are contributing to the increasing prevalence of prediabetes in young people.

Not only are children with obesity at greater risk for prediabetes and diabetes, but they may suffer bone and joint problems, *sleep apnea* (periods of stopping breathing during sleep that lead to extreme fatigue during the day), and social and psychological problems. In Chapter 11, we offer specific advice about prediabetes and obesity in children and adolescents.

Prediabetes and diabetes in older adults

Older adults, those aged 65 and above, are at the highest risk for developing elevated blood sugar and diabetes. According to the latest CDC data in the US about 29 percent of people aged 65 and older have diabetes, and an additional 48.8 percent have prediabetes. This data means that nearly four out of five older adults in the United States are affected by one of these conditions, and only about one in five have neither.

When prediabetes and diabetes are combined with other common health challenges in older age such as heart disease, reduced kidney function, and cognitive decline, the result can be significant illness, the need for multiple medications, and a higher risk of complications that require ongoing medical care. Managing blood sugar is therefore an important part of maintaining health and independence for many older adults.

REMEMBER

Prediabetes in the elderly is reversible just as it is in children, adolescents, and adults. Reversing the condition may be more difficult because of the reduced ability to exercise and the tendency to eat a less healthful diet, but it's never too late to prevent and reverse prediabetes.

Considering the Costs

The health and economic burden of elevated blood sugar is enormous and continues to grow. In 2022, the total annual cost of diabetes in the US reached $412.9 billion, including $306.6 billion in direct medical costs and $106.3 billion in indirect costs such as lost productivity. About one in every four healthcare dollars in the US is now spent on caring for people with diabetes. Beyond these financial figures, there are also significant personal costs: individuals and families often face ongoing physical challenges, emotional stress, and disruptions to daily life as they manage the complications and demands of living with diabetes and prediabetes.

Actual health costs

Most of the costs of diabetes and prediabetes are for treating the complications which include:

>> Eye disease possibly leading to blindness

>> Kidney disease possibly leading to kidney failure

>> Nerve disease possibly leading to severe pain or amputation

>> Heart disease and arterial disease possibly leading to heart attacks, strokes, or severe leg pain

REMEMBER

The fact is that the top three complications will *never occur* if prediabetes is reversed or never allowed to occur in the first place. Stopping prediabetes in its tracks is preventive medicine. Unfortunately, health insurance companies are willing to spend the thousands needed for treating the end results of disease but won't spend the much smaller sums needed to prevent the complications in the first place.

The Diabetes Prevention Program shows that preventive methods such as diet and exercise delay the development of Type 2 diabetes by an average of eleven years and reduces the number of new cases of diabetes by 20 percent.

According to recent estimates in the US, people with diabetes have medical expenditures 2.6 times higher than those without the condition. Among Medicare beneficiaries aged 65 or older with Type 2 diabetes, the median cost associated with diabetes complications is nearly $5,900 per person each year. Up to 64 percent of a person's lifetime medical costs with diabetes are spent on managing these complications.

Other economic costs

The indirect costs of diabetes and prediabetes are also substantial. These include lost productivity, higher disability rates, and increased taxes to cover public health expenditures. For example, indirect costs — such as missed work and reduced ability to work — add more than $90 billion to the national burden in the US each year. The societal cost savings from effective prevention programs are estimated to be as high as $8,800 per person.

Industries across the economy, from manufacturing to services, are affected by these costs. The high price of diabetes-related care is a significant challenge for employers, health insurers, and public programs such as Medicare and Medicaid.

Social costs

People who suffer blindness or kidney failure can't work at the level of people without these conditions, so much of their productivity is lost. Sometimes these complications — and the heart disease that is so much worse with diabetes — lead to an early death, so the losses from diabetes also affect entire families.

Because prediabetes and Type 2 diabetes are now being seen so often in children and adolescents, we can expect that people will develop complications at much younger ages. People who should be in the prime of their lives will instead be suffering illness and premature death.

The goal of this book is to show you that such a path isn't inevitable and that these costs can be avoided. By reading this book you can begin finding out how to walk the road back to health.

Chapter **2**

Suspecting Prediabetes in Yourself or a Loved One

You gained a few pounds over the years. You don't have the energy you used to have. Your mother has diabetes, and you have been reading about this condition called prediabetes so you want to know whether you may have it. In this chapter you find everything you need to know to tell whether you or a loved one may have prediabetes or diabetes. If, after reading this chapter, your suspicion is confirmed, the next step is to see a doctor to get yourself tested.

Taking a Risk Quiz

You don't need to wait for a lab test to start thinking about your risk for prediabetes. In fact, a number of simple online tools are now available to help you assess your personal risk in just a few minutes, using information you probably already know about yourself. One of the most trusted is the American Diabetes Association (ADA) Diabetes Risk Test, developed in collaboration with the US Centers for Disease Control and Prevention (CDC).

This short questionnaire doesn't diagnose prediabetes or diabetes, but it gives you a reliable estimate of how likely it is that you already have prediabetes and should be tested by your healthcare provider.

The ADA tool looks at seven key risk factors:

>> Age

>> Sex assigned at birth

>> Family history of diabetes

>> History of high blood pressure

>> Physical activity levels

>> History of gestational diabetes (for women)

>> Body weight and height (used to calculate BMI)

Each answer is assigned a particular score, and when you total them up, you get a number between 0 and 11. A score of 5 or higher suggests you're at increased risk of having prediabetes or Type 2 diabetes and should talk to a healthcare provider about getting tested. The good news is that finding out early gives you the best possible chance to take action and prevent or delay diabetes.

You can take the test online at www.diabetes.org/risk-test or fill it out on paper — it takes just a minute or two.

Different countries use different risk assessment tools which may differ slightly. For example, in the UK, the Q-Diabetes score is commonly used, while in parts of Europe, the FINDRISC (Finnish Diabetes Risk Score) is widely used to identify people at risk of Type 2 diabetes and prediabetes.

TIP

If you're unsure of your weight in pounds or height in inches, many versions of the tool now support metric units (kilograms and centimeters), making it easy to use wherever you live.

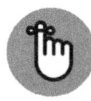

REMEMBER

Even if you score low on the ADA risk test, it doesn't guarantee that you do not have prediabetes or may develop it later. The only way of knowing for sure is with a blood test. Being aware of how your lifestyle affects your long-term health is still important. Staying active, eating a good diet, and maintaining a healthy weight can reduce your risk of prediabetes and many other chronic conditions.

Identifying Key Risk Factors That You Can Control

There's not much you can do about your age. But you can alter all the other risk factors that promote prediabetes and diabetes. In this section, we introduce these factors and point you to the chapters later in the book that give specific advice on how to affect them.

Understanding the best prediabetes diet

A truly effective prediabetes diet should also offer broad health benefits that go beyond blood sugar control. It should help lower the risk of chronic diseases commonly linked to prediabetes and diabetes, such as heart disease and high blood pressure, as well as other conditions such as dementia and cancers. Importantly, the best diet is also one that is enjoyable and satisfying, making it easier to maintain as a lifelong habit. It should also be environmentally sustainable, supporting both personal and planetary health.

While choosing the right carbohydrate foods is especially important, because these are broken down directly into glucose, other aspects of the diet matter as well. The types of fats and proteins you eat, along with vitamins, minerals, and other micronutrients, all play roles in how your body manages blood sugar. The way foods are combined in meals, how they are prepared, and even the timing of eating can influence blood glucose responses. The interaction between diet and the gut microbiome, the trillions of bacteria and other microbes in our digestive tract, also affects inflammation, metabolism, and glucose handling. Many foods contain bioactive compounds such as polyphenols, which have antioxidant and anti-inflammatory effects that can support metabolic health and reduce cardiovascular risk.

One dietary pattern that stands out for prediabetes and diabetes is the Mediterranean diet. This way of eating emphasizes vegetables, fruits, whole grains, legumes, nuts, extra virgin olive oil, moderate amounts of fish and poultry, only limited red meat and sweets, and excluding ultra processed foods altogether. The Mediterranean diet has been named the best overall diet for diabetes and prediabetes for several years running by the annual *U.S. News & World Report* panel of nutrition experts. Decades of research, including clinical trials and large population studies show that this approach improves blood sugar control, supports weight management, and reduces the risk of heart disease and stroke. Its focus on fresh, nutrient-rich foods and healthy fats makes it both effective and enjoyable, and its flexibility helps people sustain it over the long term.

The best diet for prediabetes is not about strict rules or deprivation, but about making informed, enjoyable, and sustainable choices that support your overall health and well-being. Later chapters explore the evidence behind different dietary patterns and offer practical guidance for putting these principles into action.

Evaluating the best prediabetes lifestyle

The best lifestyle for prediabetes is one that supports healthy blood sugar control, potentially reversing the diagnosis, reduces the risk of developing Type 2 diabetes, and promotes overall well-being. Adopting such a lifestyle goes beyond just diet; it involves a combination of regular physical activity, effective stress management, restorative sleep, and maintaining a healthy weight. These habits work together to improve the body's sensitivity to insulin, help regulate glucose levels, and lower the risk of related health problems.

A well-rounded lifestyle for prediabetes should be enjoyable and sustainable, fitting naturally into your daily routine. Regular movement, whether it's brisk walking, cycling, swimming, or strength training, helps your muscles use glucose more effectively and can make a significant difference in blood sugar control. Managing stress through relaxation techniques, hobbies, or mindfulness practices can also have a positive impact, as chronic stress can raise blood sugar and reduce the effectiveness of insulin, the hormone that regulates glucose management. Prioritizing good sleep is equally important, because poor sleep is linked to higher glucose levels and increased diabetes risk.

Other key elements include avoiding smoking and moderating alcohol intake. These choices not only support blood sugar health but also reduce the risk of heart disease, high blood pressure, and other conditions often associated with prediabetes. The best lifestyle is one that feels rewarding, is flexible enough to adapt to life's changes, and can be maintained over the long term.

Focusing on your weight

The relationship between body weight and prediabetes is well established, with higher body weight, especially in the overweight or obese range significantly increasing the risk of developing prediabetes and progressing to Type 2 diabetes. One common way to assess whether someone is in a healthy weight range is by calculating Body Mass Index (BMI) which takes into account a person's height. BMI is a simple formula: weight in pounds divided by height in inches squared $\times$ 703 (or kilograms divided by height in meters squared).

According to standard categories, a BMI below 18.5 is considered underweight, 18.5 to 24.9 is normal weight, 25 to 29.9 is overweight, and 30 or above is classified as obese. Research shows that as BMI increases, so does the risk of developing problems with blood sugar regulation, prediabetes, and eventually Type 2 diabetes.

As BMI rises, particularly when this increase reflects higher levels of body fat, it is often associated with a cluster of health problems known as *metabolic syndrome*. Metabolic syndrome is a combination of risk factors, including increased waist circumference, high blood pressure, abnormal cholesterol levels, and elevated blood glucose, which together raise the risk of heart disease, stroke, and diabetes. When there is more body fat, especially around the abdomen, the body's ability to use insulin efficiently is reduced. This means the hormone insulin becomes less effective at moving glucose from the bloodstream into the cells, making it harder to keep blood glucose within a healthy range.

However, BMI has important limitations. It does not distinguish between muscle and fat, so very muscular individuals such as athletes or rugby players may have a high BMI but low body fat and excellent metabolic health. In older adults, a slightly higher BMI may not carry the same risks, as it can reflect greater bone density or muscle mass rather than excess fat. In fact, some studies suggest that in the elderly, being in the overweight category may even be associated with lower mortality compared to being underweight or at the lower end of the normal range.

Beyond total body weight, the distribution and type of fat are crucial for health, particularly when it comes to prediabetes and cardiovascular risk. *Visceral fat,* which is stored deep within the abdomen and surrounds vital organs such as the liver and intestines, is especially harmful. Unlike subcutaneous fat (the fat just under the skin), visceral fat is metabolically active and releases inflammatory substances that contribute to higher blood pressure, difficulties with blood sugar regulation, and increased risk of heart disease, stroke, and certain cancers. Waist circumference is a practical way to estimate visceral fat: a waist measurement above 37 inches (about 94 cm) for men or 31.5 inches (about 80 cm) for women suggests a higher risk. People who carry more weight around their abdomen ("apple-shaped" body) are at greater risk than those who carry weight around their hips and thighs ("pear-shaped" body).

It's important to note that while higher BMI is associated with greater risk of prediabetes and diabetes across all dietary patterns, certain eating habits can help offset this risk. For example, following a Mediterranean diet rich in vegetables, fruits, whole grains, healthy fats, and lean proteins has been shown to reduce the risk of developing diabetes, even in those with higher BMI. This element suggests that lifestyle factors, including diet quality and physical activity, play a key role in modifying the risk associated with body weight.

While maintaining a healthy weight is an important part of preventing and managing prediabetes, it's equally important to consider body composition, fat distribution, and lifestyle habits. Focusing on reducing visceral fat through balanced nutrition and regular physical activity can significantly improve the body's ability to manage blood sugar and lower the risk of progression to diabetes and related health problems.

Getting up and moving

Regular physical activity is one of the most effective ways to prevent or reverse prediabetes and help stop its progression to Type 2 diabetes. Exercise improves the body's sensitivity to insulin, allowing glucose to move more efficiently from the bloodstream into the muscles, where it can be used for energy. This not only helps regulate blood glucose levels but also supports weight management, reduces inflammation, and lowers the risk of cardiovascular disease which are all important goals for anyone with prediabetes.

Current recommendations from leading health authorities, including the US Department of Health and Human Services (HHS) and the American Diabetes Association (ADA), emphasize that adults should aim for at least 150 minutes per week of moderate-intensity aerobic activity, such as brisk walking, cycling, or swimming. This exercise can be spread throughout the week in sessions of 20–30 minutes at a time. For those who prefer more vigorous activities, 75 minutes per week of higher-intensity exercise, such as jogging or fast cycling, provides similar benefits. In addition to aerobic activity, muscle-strengthening exercises such as resistance training with weights, bands, or bodyweight are recommended at least two days per week, as they further improve glucose regulation and overall metabolic health.

Importantly, even small amounts of physical activity are better than none, and the benefits increase with greater frequency, duration, or intensity. Recent research also supports the value of shorter, *higher-intensity interval training* (HIIT), which can improve insulin efficiency and blood glucose control in less time. For example, brief bursts of intense exercise, such as cycling sprints or stair climbing, performed a few times a week, have been shown to produce meaningful improvements in glucose metabolism, even in people with busy schedules.

TIP

For older adults or those with mobility challenges, any movement counts. Activities such as walking, gardening, or gentle stretching can help maintain muscle strength, balance, and flexibility, reducing the risk of falls and supporting independence. The key is to find activities that are enjoyable and sustainable, making it easier to incorporate movement into daily life.

Regular exercise is a cornerstone of prediabetes management. Whether through structured workouts or everyday activities, moving more and sitting less can make a significant difference in blood sugar control and overall health. Later chapters provide practical tips and strategies to help you get started and stay motivated, regardless of your current fitness level.

Dealing with stress

Stress is recognized as an important factor in both prediabetes and diabetes. When the body encounters stress, it releases hormones such as adrenaline and cortisol. These stress hormones are part of the body's natural "fight or flight" response, helping to increase alertness and physical readiness. However, one of the side effects of these hormones is an increase in blood glucose levels, as the body mobilizes energy to respond to perceived threats. Over time, frequent or chronic stress can contribute to difficulties in maintaining healthy blood sugar control.

In addition to its direct physiological effects, stress can also influence lifestyle habits that are important for managing prediabetes. During periods of stress, you may find it more challenging to maintain regular physical activity, follow a balanced diet, or keep up with other healthy routines. This can further complicate efforts to regulate blood glucose and overall health.

Effective strategies for managing stress may include relaxation techniques, mindfulness practices, regular physical activity, and seeking social support. Finding constructive ways to cope with stress can play a valuable role in supporting both emotional well-being and metabolic health. Later chapters explore practical approaches to stress management in greater detail, while providing tools and guidance to help reduce the impact of stress on daily life and blood glucose regulation.

Getting enough sleep

Adequate, high-quality sleep is increasingly recognized as being important in maintaining healthy blood glucose regulation and reducing the risk of developing prediabetes and progressing from prediabetes to Type 2 diabetes. Research shows that consistently getting too little sleep, typically less than 7 hours per night for adults, can disrupt important hormonal and metabolic processes that control blood glucose. Poor or insufficient sleep is linked to higher levels of stress hormones, increased appetite, and reduced insulin efficiency, all of which can make it harder for the body to keep blood glucose within a healthy range.

Sleep deprivation can also contribute to weight gain and increased cravings for high-carbohydrate and energy-dense foods. Disrupted sleep patterns, such as those caused by shift work or frequent night-time awakenings, have been associated with greater risk of developing reduced insulin efficiency and *metabolic syndrome* — a cluster of conditions including increased obesity, high blood pressure, elevated blood glucose and high cholesterol, which is discussed further in Chapter 5. Over time, these effects can make it more difficult to manage prediabetes and increase the likelihood of developing Type 2 diabetes and related complications.

Prioritizing good sleep hygiene is an important part of a healthy lifestyle for anyone with prediabetes. This includes maintaining a regular sleep schedule, creating a restful sleep environment, limiting exposure to screens and bright lights before bedtime, and avoiding caffeine or heavy meals in the evening. Regular physical activity and stress management techniques can also support better sleep quality. By making sleep a priority, individuals can help support their body's ability to regulate blood glucose and protect long-term metabolic health.

Understanding How Prediabetes and Diabetes Develop

When your metabolism is normal, your blood glucose is controlled within a narrow range, from a low of about 70 mg/dl (3.9 mmol/L) when you are fasting to a high of about 139 mg/dl (7.7 mmol/L) one hour after eating. This section explains how a healthy body keeps such a tight grip on glucose and what goes wrong when that grip slips.

Keeping glucose under control

Insulin is a *hormone* (a chemical made in an organ, in this case the pancreas) that enters the bloodstream and affects cells throughout the body. Insulin opens these cells so glucose can enter and provide the energy needed by your muscles, your fat, and many other tissues. Without insulin, glucose in your bloodstream can't be utilized.

REMEMBER

Insulin permits the building up of muscle, fat, and other tissues. In this sense it is the builder hormone. You can't build your body without insulin. It also provides for storage of excess glucose in the form of glycogen so that it is ready to quickly provide energy as the glucose level falls. You do not live long without insulin.

Insulin sensitivity and insulin resistance are terms used to describe how efficiently your body's cells respond to insulin. When you are *insulin sensitive,* your cells readily respond to insulin's signal, allowing glucose to move easily from your bloodstream into your muscles, fat, and other tissues for energy or storage. This helps keep your blood glucose tightly regulated. *Insulin resistance,* on the other hand, means your cells do not respond as well to insulin's signal. As a result, your pancreas must produce more insulin to achieve the same effect, and over time, this can lead to higher blood glucose levels and eventually to prediabetes or diabetes.

The good news is that insulin sensitivity is not fixed — it can be improved with healthy lifestyle choices. Regular physical activity, such as brisk walking, cycling, or strength training, helps your muscles use glucose more effectively and increases insulin sensitivity. A balanced diet that emphasizes whole grains, vegetables, lean proteins, healthy fats, and limits added sugars and highly processed foods also supports better insulin action. Maintaining a healthy weight, getting enough sleep, and managing stress are additional factors that can help reduce insulin resistance. By making these changes, you can help your body use insulin more efficiently and keep your blood glucose in a healthy range.

REMEMBER

A combination of your genetic predisposition, age, body fat, and lifestyle choices including your diet and the amount of exercise you enjoy, all contribute to how sensitive or resistant your body is to insulin and how efficiently your blood glucose levels are managed.

Losing control of glucose

With increasing insulin resistance, blood glucose levels rise to levels of prediabetes, and if left unchecked, may well increase beyond this range to levels which meet the criteria for a diagnosis of diabetes. When the glucose rises to 180 mg/dl (10 mmol/L) in the blood, your kidneys can no longer return all the glucose to the blood and it starts to spill into your urine. You begin to develop some annoying complications. Because the glucose in prediabetes can rise as high as 199 mg/dl, you can have these complications even in prediabetes. They include

>> Frequent urination and thirst because the glucose in the urine pulls water out of your body and fills your bladder, making you want to urinate more often. As you lose water you get thirsty.

>> Fatigue because the cells are not getting the energy they need.

>> Persistent vaginal infection in women because there is some spilling of glucose over the vaginal tissues, and yeast loves a sweet surface to grow on. There is itching, burning, an abnormal discharge, and sometimes an odor.

As the insulin in your body declines further or becomes even less effective, you start to develop long-term complications, especially heart disease, eye disease, kidney disease, and nerve disease. At this point, you have diabetes. You can still prevent these unpleasant complications by lifestyle changes and perhaps medication, but isn't it so much better never to get to this stage?

Appreciating prediabetes is a problem

Prediabetes is more than just a warning sign for Type 2 diabetes, it's also an early indicator that your risk for cardiovascular disease (CVD), including heart attacks, strokes, and high blood pressure, is already on the rise. Studies show that these cardiovascular risks begin to increase during the prediabetes stage, long before blood sugar reaches the diabetic range, and become even more significant if diabetes develops and remains poorly controlled.

A central process in the development of cardiovascular disease is *atherosclerosis,* which occurs when the inner walls of the arteries become damaged and inflamed, leading to the gradual build-up of fatty deposits called *plaques.* Over time, these plaques can narrow or block arteries, restricting blood flow to the heart, brain, and other vital organs, and are the underlying cause of most heart attacks and strokes.

The link between prediabetes, diabetes, and atherosclerosis centers on the harmful effects of elevated blood sugar on blood vessels. Even moderately high glucose levels, sustained over time, can injure the delicate lining of the arteries (the endothelium). One important culprit is the formation of *advanced glycation end-products* (AGEs) — harmful compounds created when excess glucose attaches to proteins and fats in the body. AGEs promote inflammation, increase oxidative stress, and make blood vessels stiffer and more vulnerable to blockage, all of which accelerate the development of cardiovascular disease.

High blood sugar also makes the blood more likely to clot and reduces the arteries' ability to relax and adapt to changes in blood flow, further increasing the risk of cardiovascular complications even before diabetes is fully established.

As HbA1c levels rise from the prediabetes range into mild diabetes and then possibly into poorly controlled diabetes, the risk of cardiovascular damage climbs steadily. This is why recognizing prediabetes early and making lifestyle changes to improve blood sugar control is so important, not just to prevent diabetes, but also to protect your heart and circulatory system for the long term.

Seeking a Medical Diagnosis

Earlier in this chapter we provide a risk quiz that you can take if you think you may have prediabetes. Obviously, the quiz can leave you with a large amount of suspicion but not a definite diagnosis. For a diagnosis, you need to see a doctor.

Healthcare systems differ worldwide, but the core principles of effective prediabetes care remain consistent. Care should be accurate, evidence-based, clearly communicated, and tailored to the individual. Whether you access care through a national health service, private insurance, or local clinics, the aim is to identify prediabetes early and provide structured support to better regulate your blood glucose, reverse prediabetes, reduce your likelihood of developing Type 2 diabetes, decrease the risk of developing chronic diseases including cardiovascular disease such as stroke and heart attack, and to live a long and healthy life.

Who to see and what to expect

In most countries, a primary care doctor — often called a general practitioner (GP) — family physician, or internal medicine doctor, can diagnose and manage prediabetes. These professionals are trained to interpret test results, assess overall health risks, and create a personalized plan to help you lower your risk. If your case is more complex or your blood glucose levels continue to rise despite initial efforts, your doctor may refer you to a specialist such as an *endocrinologist* (a doctor specializing in hormone and metabolic disorders) or a *diabetologist* (a physician with advanced training in diabetes management).

At your appointment, you can expect tests such as HbA1c, fasting blood glucose, or an oral glucose tolerance test. Other assessments may include blood pressure, cholesterol, kidney function, and measurements of weight, height, and body mass index (BMI). These tests help your healthcare provider understand your current health status and guide further recommendations. In addition, your doctor may use a 10-year cardiovascular risk assessment tool — such as QRISK in the UK, the ASCVD Risk Estimator in the US, or SCORE2 in Europe — to estimate your likelihood of developing heart disease or stroke over the next decade. These algorithms take into account factors such as age, sex, blood pressure, cholesterol, smoking status, and medical history including prediabetes or diabetes, providing a comprehensive picture of your cardiovascular risk and helping inform decisions about preventive treatments and lifestyle changes.

Building a support program for lifestyle change

Managing prediabetes effectively requires more than brief advice from a doctor. Evidence shows that structured, intensive lifestyle programs are far more successful at supporting lasting change and reducing the risk of diabetes. In the UK, the NHS Diabetes Prevention Program (NHS DPP) offers a national, evidence-based service for people at high risk of Type 2 diabetes in the UK. Participants are referred by their GP and receive group-based, intensive lifestyle counselling focused on weight loss, physical activity, and healthy eating. Research has shown that referral to the NHS DPP leads to improved blood glucose control, weight loss, and reductions in cardiovascular risk factors.

In the United States, the Centers for Disease Control and Prevention (CDC) runs the National Diabetes Prevention Program (National DPP), which provides access to affordable, high-quality lifestyle change programs across the country. These programs are delivered by trained lifestyle coaches and include group sessions, goal setting, self-monitoring, and ongoing support to help participants achieve and maintain healthy habits. Both the British and American DPPs are based on the landmark research, which demonstrate that lifestyle interventions can reduce the risk of developing diabetes by up to 58 percent over three years.

Engaging a broader support team

Beyond national programs, many people benefit from building a wider support network. This support may include working with a registered dietitian or nutritionist for personalized dietary advice, a physical therapist or exercise professional for safe and effective physical activity plans, or a health coach for motivation and accountability. Some also offer access to diabetes prevention educators or peer support groups, which can provide encouragement and shared experiences. Research suggests that group-based interventions and social support can enhance motivation and lead to greater improvements in health outcomes.

Personal trainers or fitness instructors can help tailor exercise routines to your abilities and preferences, while community-based classes can make it easier to stay engaged. For those with barriers to attending in-person sessions, many programs now offer remote or digital options, increasing accessibility and flexibility. Enjoying the exercise you do is important.

Counsellors, mental health experts, or other complementary wellbeing practitioners can help with issues or depression, anxiety or stress which may be preventing you managing your health.

It is important to make sure that any practitioner is appropriately trained and registered with a professional standards or regulatory organization.

When specialist advice is needed

If prediabetes progresses such as when blood glucose levels rise into the diabetic range or complications develop, specialist input may become necessary. An endocrinologist or diabetologist can provide advanced diagnostic testing, initiate or adjust medication, and manage complex cases, including those with other medical conditions or early complications such as nerve, eye, or kidney changes. Referral to a diabetes specialist nurse or a multidisciplinary diabetes care team may also be recommended for more comprehensive support.

The importance of ongoing support and follow-up

Prediabetes is a dynamic condition, and ongoing support is crucial for long-term success. Regular follow-up appointments enable your healthcare provider to monitor your progress, repeat key tests, and adjust your care plan as needed. If you encounter challenges such as difficulty maintaining lifestyle changes or new health issues don't hesitate to seek additional help. National and local programs, as well as digital health tools, can provide continued guidance and motivation.

The most important measurement of success is with the regular testing of HbA1c. This test provides a clear picture of your average blood glucose over the previous two to three months and is an excellent way to monitor your progress over time. The goal is to reduce your HbA1c level to below the prediabetes threshold of 42 mmol/mol (expressed as 6.0 percent in the US) and to prevent it from rising above 48 mmol/mol (expressed as 6.5 percent in the US), which is the cutoff for diabetes. Regular HbA1c testing allows you and your healthcare provider to track improvements, adjust your care plan as needed, and stay focused on long-term prevention.

Ultimately, the most effective care for prediabetes is built on partnership, clear communication, and a supportive environment. By making use of structured programs, engaging a multidisciplinary team, and staying connected to your healthcare provider, you can take meaningful steps to reduce your risk of diabetes and improve your overall health.

Chapter **3**

Tracking the Transition from Prediabetes to Diabetes

edically speaking, the distinction between prediabetes and diabetes is designated by going from one level of blood glucose to another, usually defined by your HbA1C — the blood test that shows your average level of blood glucose over the past two to three months, rising above 48 mmol/mol (or 6.5 percent). But in real life, the division between the two conditions is not so sharp. People with blood glucose levels that are persistently high but not quite in the diabetic range sometimes have complications that are supposed to be found only in diabetes, such as eye disease and nerve disease. There is also an increased risk above normal of cardiovascular diseases such as stroke and heart disease, dementia and kidney disease. (So, your goal should be not only to avoid going from prediabetes to diabetes but also to keep your blood glucose in the normal range.)

REMEMBER

When prediabetes progresses, it leads specifically to Type 2 diabetes. Type 1 diabetes is a separate condition that typically develops suddenly and is not caused by the slow, gradual loss of insulin regulation seen in prediabetes and Type 2 diabetes.

The risk of getting diabetes is as much as *ten times greater* if you have prediabetes than if you have normal blood glucose levels. So, if you suspect you have prediabetes, you need to act now to make sure it doesn't become diabetes.

We start the chapter by talking about the signs and symptoms that should alert you that you may be making the transition into diabetes. We then introduce the short-term and long-term complications that arise when you become a person with diabetes.

With rare exceptions, you *can* prevent the transition from prediabetes to diabetes.

Turning Prediabetes into Diabetes

In the effort to prevent prediabetes from progressing to diabetes, several persistent roadblocks remain:

» **Insurance coverage:** In many countries, health insurance companies still do not consistently pay for lifestyle-focused treatments, such as sessions with dietitians, physical trainers, psychologists, or social workers. However, progress has been made in some regions. For example, the CDC's National Diabetes Prevention Program in the US and the NHS Diabetes Prevention Program in the UK are now covered by Medicare and the NHS, respectively, offering structured lifestyle support to those at high risk.

» **Medications:** Currently no FDA-approved medications exist specifically for treating impaired fasting glucose or impaired glucose tolerance (the main forms of prediabetes). Metformin is sometimes recommended off-label for people at particularly high risk, but it is not officially approved for prediabetes.

» **Variation in medical practice:** While there is now broad agreement among major organizations such as the American Diabetes Association (ADA), International Diabetes Federation (IDF), and NICE (The UK's National Institute for Health and Care Excellence) on the importance of lifestyle intervention as first-line management, some variation in clinical practice remains.

» **Setting targets:** There are no universally agreed-upon, definitive targets for weight, blood glucose, blood pressure, or cholesterol that guarantee diabetes prevention. However, guidelines do recommend aiming for modest weight loss (typically 5–10 percent of body weight), blood pressure below 130/80 mmHg, LDL cholesterol within guideline-specific targets, and HbA1c below the prediabetes threshold.

>> **Advocacy remains important:** Expanding insurance coverage for preventive services and supporting research into new treatment options can help more people access effective care. Setting practical, evidence-based goals, even if they are approximations, can help guide both patients and clinicians in monitoring progress.

Despite these challenges, people continue to move from prediabetes to diabetes every day. The transition is defined by specific laboratory criteria. Diabetes is diagnosed when a fasting blood glucose result is 126 mg/dL (7.0 mmol/L) or higher, or when your blood glucose two hours after consuming 75 grams of glucose is 200 mg/dL (11.1 mmol/L) or higher, confirmed on two separate occasions. Increasingly, however, the most commonly used diagnostic criterion is the HbA1c test, with a value of 48 mmol/mol (6.5 percent) or above indicating diabetes. HbA1c is widely used because it reflects average blood glucose over the previous two to three months and does not require fasting.

But before you even go to the doctor and have a blood test, you can look for these clues that you're crossing the line:

>> You are gaining weight.

>> You have decreased your level of exercise or are injured and can't exercise.

>> You urinate frequently and often feel thirsty.

>> You feel fatigued.

>> You are a woman who is getting frequent vaginal infections with yeast or some other organism.

So, what actually happens to tip prediabetes into diabetes? Nothing very earth-shaking. Just getting a little older can lower your insulin sensitivity so that your body's insulin can't keep your fasting glucose level under 126 mg/dL or your HbA1c level to below the diabetes threshold of 48 mmol/mol (6.5 percent).

Or allowing yourself to gain a few pounds can do it. Reducing your physical activity can result in a rise in your blood glucose to 126 mg/dL or higher, especially if you were doing vigorous physical exercise before and can't now because of an injury or illness. If several of these factors are happening at the same time, which is often the case, the likelihood that prediabetes will turn into diabetes is even greater.

People with either impaired fasting glucose or impaired glucose tolerance (see Chapter 1) convert to diabetes at the rate of about 8 to 10 percent per year. However, for people who have *both* conditions, the rate is much higher.

Recognizing Short-Term Effects of Diabetes

Symptoms that develop when diabetes occurs are divided into short-term and long-term complications. This chapter offers an overview so you know what you're trying to avoid.

Short-term effects result from persistent elevations of blood glucose or sudden falls in blood glucose. They are immediately treatable, and the abnormality is reversed as long as the rise or fall in blood glucose doesn't recur. These short-term complications can occur at any stage in the course of diabetes, not just at the beginning. But as patients become more familiar with their disease, these effects usually occur less often.

Handling hypoglycemia

Hypoglycemia means low blood glucose. There is no exact level of blood glucose that defines hypoglycemia because some people develop symptoms at 70 mg/dL (3.9 mmol/L) and others are still comfortable at that blood level but have symptoms at 60 mg/dL (3.3 mmol/L). Hypoglycemia does not result from the diabetes itself but from the drugs that we use to treat high blood glucose.

Symptoms

Some of the important symptoms that suggest hypoglycemia are:

>> Hunger

>> Sweating

>> Mental confusion or even coma

>> Rapid heartbeat

>> Headache

>> Visual disturbances such as double vision

Triggers

Here are some of the substances and circumstances that can bring on hypoglycemia either by themselves or when you have taken a drug to lower your blood glucose:

>> *Sulfonylureas,* which are drugs taken by mouth to lower glucose with names such as Orinase, Diabinase, and glyburide

>> Insulin, usually taken by injection

>> Aspirin or other salicylates

>> Alcohol

>> Too little food for the glucose-lowering drug in your body

>> Too much exercise for the glucose-lowering drug in your body

Simple treatments

Most hypoglycemia is mild and responds to simple measures. You should be better within 20 minutes after taking one these treatments:

>> Two sugar cubes

>> Two or three glucose tablets

>> Six ounces of a sugary soft drink

>> Eight ounces of milk

>> Four ounces of orange juice

Managing ketoacidosis

Ketoacidosis isn't common in someone with Type 2 diabetes, but it occasionally happens, especially when the person has a severe infection or great physical stress. What happens is that the blood glucose rises very high, sometimes to 500 or 600 mg/dL (27.8 to 33.3 mmol/L). No glucose is getting into cells so the body turns to fat for energy. As fat breaks down, it produces a lot of acidic breakdown products. The large amount of sugar in the blood can't be held back by the kidneys and flows into the urine, pulling a lot of body water with it. The person becomes dehydrated and *acidotic* (meaning they have an abnormal increase of acids in their blood), leading to nausea and vomiting, which further depletes the body not only of water but of minerals like potassium.

WARNING

You may notice that you have some symptoms of ketoacidosis and begin to suspect that you have this complication. But that diagnosis is best made by a doctor, preferably in the hospital where you can begin treatment at once.

Symptoms

Ketoacidosis is associated with many symptoms, which make it fairly easy to realize what is happening. Among them are:

>> Nausea and vomiting.

>> Rapid breathing known as *Kussmaul breathing*. Your body is attempting to reduce the acid in your blood by blowing it off through the lungs. Your breath has a fruity smell due to the acetone from the fat.

>> Extreme tiredness and drowsiness because the blood that circulates in your brain is thick like syrup and is missing essential substances.

>> Weakness due to lack of fuel (glucose), which is elevated in the blood but can't get into your cells.

Signs

Unlike symptoms, which you can notice yourself, *signs* are the details that are observed by other people, particularly your doctor when you reach the hospital. The signs of ketoacidosis are:

>> High blood glucose, usually more than 300 mg/dL (16.6 mmol/L)

>> High levels of acid in your blood

>> High levels of *ketones* (the products of the breakdown of fats) in your blood and urine

>> Dry skin and tongue consistent with dehydration

>> Deficiency of potassium in your body

>> Acetone smell on your breath

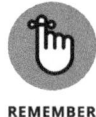

REMEMBER

Another situation, when you aren't sick, may cause you to have a lot of ketones in your blood and urine. That's when you go on a diet and your fat cells begin to break down. Your glucose levels are likely to be just fine in this situation.

Treatment

Treatment of ketoacidosis is done by a physician in the hospital. The doctor gives you insulin to make up for the lack of active insulin in your body, replaces lost potassium, and gives you a lot of intravenous fluids to rehydrate your body.

The treatments are all done very rapidly, and sometimes the patient is okay in 36 hours. However, if the ketoacidosis is brought on by a severe infection or other trauma, it may resist treatment and even end in death.

Dealing with the hyperosmolar syndrome

People who have this short-term complication of diabetes have some of the highest blood glucose levels. So much glucose is in the blood that it is literally like maple syrup. As you can imagine, your blood vessels were not meant to carry maple syrup.

This complication, which is now sometimes called *hyperosmolar hyperglycemic state* often occurs in elderly people who were not even known to have diabetes. They may be at home or in a nursing home where they are not carefully monitored, and they become dehydrated. If they develop nausea, vomiting, or diarrhea, they may end up with even more dehydration.

The elderly also have reduced kidney function. While a younger kidney begins to leak glucose into the urine and thus outside the body at a blood level of 180 mg/dL (10 mmol/L), the older kidney does not start to leak glucose until a higher blood level is reached. If the body is already dehydrated, the reduction in the volume of blood makes it even harder for the kidneys to rid the body of glucose. So, the blood glucose rises even higher.

As the body becomes further dehydrated, the blood pressure starts to fall, and the patient gets weaker and weaker. They also become confused. Their mental state declines until they become comatose.

The patient does not become very acidotic in this condition, unlike with ketoacidosis, because they have enough insulin to prevent the breakdown of fat. There is no Kussmaul breathing and no smell of acetone on the breath.

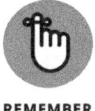

REMEMBER

Severe infection and the failure to take insulin are other causes of hyperosmolar syndrome, but dehydration due to reduced water intake, nausea, vomiting, and diarrhea is the most frequent cause.

Symptoms

These patients have symptoms that are discovered fairly easily if anyone is paying attention to them. Among the most important are:

>> Frequent urination

>> Thirst

>> Weakness

>> Leg cramps

>> Sunken eyeballs and rapid pulse

>> Decreased mental awareness leading to coma

The key sign of this condition is a blood glucose level of 600 or even higher.

Treatment

Hyperosmolar syndrome is a medical emergency just like ketoacidosis. The patient is taken to the intensive care unit (ICU) of the hospital where the emphasis is on replacing fluids and minerals that are missing, such as potassium, sodium, and chloride. Surprisingly, very little insulin is required. As the minerals and fluid are replaced, the glucose rapidly falls. However, if the problem was initiated by a severe infection or injury, these issues must be treated for the patient to recover.

Dealing with Severe, Long-Term Complications

These long-term problems, which often occur after ten or more years of poor control of the blood glucose, include:

>> Eye disease, which may lead to blindness

>> Kidney disease, which may end in kidney failure

>> Nerve disease, which can result in pain or weakness

>> Heart disease, which usually ends in a heart attack

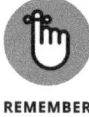

REMEMBER

These complications are not inevitable. If you reverse your prediabetes so your blood glucose is normal, or if you keep your blood glucose under control when you have diabetes or prediabetes, none of these will happen.

Viewing eye disease

Diabetes may be responsible for several different kinds of eye disease. These include:

>> **Cataracts:** These are opaque areas of the lens of the eye that can block your vision if they're large enough. Fortunately, a relatively simple operation can remove the cataract and replace it with an artificial lens that allows you to see normally.

>> **Glaucoma:** This condition involves abnormally high pressure in the eye that can damage the *optic nerve,* the nerve through which light travels to the brain, allowing us to see. Excellent medical treatment with medications is available to lower the pressure and save the sight.

>> **Diabetic retinopathy:** This condition consists of many different changes in the *retina,* the light-gathering tissue at the back of the eyeball. Some of the changes are benign, and some are dangerous to the vision, but very good treatment is available that can save your sight. Diabetic retinopathy is responsible for 15,000 to 20,000 new cases of blindness every year. But good control of the blood glucose reduces this complication by 75 percent.

Avoiding kidney disease

Your kidneys are essential for ridding your body of chemicals and toxic products of normal metabolism, as well as helping to maintain the balance of salt and water in your body. Diabetes is responsible for almost half of all new cases of kidney failure (*diabetic nephropathy*).

Diabetes affects the kidneys by damaging their filtering mechanism so they can no longer filter toxins from the blood. These poisons build up and can kill the patient if they are not removed.

One of the important ways to prevent kidney failure is to detect kidney disease in its earliest stages. Detection is done by a simple test of your urine called the *micro-albumin* test, now more commonly called the "urine albumin-to-creatinine ratio" or UACR. Normally, tiny amounts of protein escape from your blood and enter your urine. In the case of early kidney damage, the amount measured in the urine rises significantly above what is normally measured. In this situation, your doctor can prescribe a variety of medications to reverse the kidney damage. If the damage progresses to kidney failure, excellent treatments are still available in the form of kidney transplants and *dialysis,* a mechanical cleansing of the blood.

TIP

If you develop diabetes, make sure your doctor tests for microalbumin in the UACR test regularly right from the outset.

High blood glucose is not the only culprit in diabetic kidney disease. Two other abnormalities contribute: high blood pressure and high cholesterol. In treating diabetic kidney disease, you need to attack all three abnormalities. Your blood pressure should be lower than 130/80, and your cholesterol should be no higher than 200 with plenty of HDL or "good" cholesterol. Other problems, such as repeated kidney infections, can speed up the damage to the kidneys.

Detecting nerve disease

Just about any nerve in the body can be damaged by the effects of too much glucose in the blood. Careful testing may determine that as many as 70 percent of people with diabetes have nerve disease. This disease can lead to a variety of complications, which include:

>> **Disorders of sensation,** where the person can't feel a *filament,* a hair-thin piece of plastic that is touched in several places on the bottoms of the feet. This complication may lead to amputations if an injury goes undetected and a wound forms that severely damages the limb.

>> **Disorders of motion,** where the person becomes weak or loses the motion of certain muscle groups due to damage to the nerve that signals the muscle to move.

>> **Disorders of the *autonomic nerves,*** the nerves that signal the heart to pump automatically or the stomach to empty automatically or the intestine to move food and wastes along automatically.

>> **Mixed conditions** that include both loss of sensation and loss of movement.

These conditions of the nerves can make the diabetes more difficult to control. For example, if your stomach does not empty as expected, the medications that are supposed to be active as glucose is being absorbed and may act too early, causing hypoglycemia. Or physical activity, an essential part of good diabetes treatment, may be curtailed by the nerve damage.

Dodging heart disease

The heart depends on blood flow from the coronary (heart) arteries to provide oxygen and nutrition to the heart muscle. If this flow is partially obstructed, the patient may experience heart pain called *angina,* especially when the heart needs to pump harder (such as during exercise). If the flow is completely obstructed, you can have a heart attack.

REMEMBER

Coronary artery disease is the most common cause of death in patients with Type 2 diabetes. In Type 2 diabetes, coronary artery disease tends to be much more extensive than in people without diabetes, and even people with prediabetes have more coronary artery disease than people with normal levels of blood glucose.

If a heart attack occurs, the risk of death is much greater for the person with diabetes than for a person with healthy glucose levels. Someone with diabetes who has a heart attack has a 40 percent chance of dying from it. In contrast, someone with healthy glucose levels who has a heart attack has a 15 percent chance of dying. And after that first heart attack, the survival rate differs greatly between people with diabetes and people whose glucose is under control: Within five years after the heart attack, the mortality rate is 80 percent for the person with diabetes and 25 percent for someone with normal glucose levels.

Other factors promote coronary artery disease as well, whether or not diabetes is present. The most important are:

>> Obesity

>> Central fat deposition (meaning you carry your fat around the waist, not around the hips)

>> High blood pressure

>> Abnormal blood fats, especially reduced HDL (the so-called "good" cholesterol)

Any approach to the prevention of coronary artery disease in prediabetes or diabetes must address these factors as well as the blood glucose.

Sexual function

Diabetes can have a significant impact on sexual function for both men and women, due to a combination of physical, psychological, and hormonal factors. Persistently high blood glucose levels can cause damage to nerves and blood vessels, which are essential for normal sexual response. In men, this often leads to erectile dysfunction (ED), as reduced blood flow and nerve damage make it difficult to achieve or maintain an erection. Men with diabetes are also at increased risk for ejaculation problems, such as retrograde ejaculation or dry orgasm, and may experience a lower sex drive, especially if testosterone levels are low or if other risk factors such as obesity or high blood pressure are present.

Women with diabetes may experience a range of sexual health concerns, including reduced vaginal lubrication, difficulty with arousal, pain during intercourse, and a higher risk of vaginal and urinary tract infections. These issues can make sex uncomfortable or less enjoyable. Hormonal changes, nerve involvement, and the psychological effects of living with diabetes — such as stress, low self-esteem, or depression — can further contribute to reduced sexual desire and satisfaction. Both men and women may find their overall interest in sex or their ability to enjoy sexual activity affected by the demands of managing a chronic condition and by fluctuations in blood glucose levels.

It is important for people with diabetes to discuss any sexual health concerns with their healthcare provider, as many issues can be managed or treated. Addressing blood glucose control, reviewing medications, and seeking support for emotional well-being can all help improve sexual function and quality of life.

Pregnancy problems

Diabetes can add a lot of burdens to the difficulties that a woman faces during the joyous occasion of pregnancy. The problems are not only the mother's, but they extend to the growing baby.

Problems for the mother

Many mothers already know that they have diabetes before they become pregnant. If that's the case, it's up to them to achieve the best possible glucose control before becoming pregnant. When the baby is conceived during a period of poor glucose control in the mother, the probability of a congenital malformation (such as absence of part of the brain or splitting of the spinal column with paralysis in the baby) is much greater.

Some of the other problems that diabetes promotes in a pregnancy include:

>> Difficulty in conceiving a baby in the first place

>> More frequent miscarriages

>> More frequent *caesarean sections* (surgery through the abdomen to remove the baby)

>> The need for early delivery due to the large size of the baby

New cases of diabetes can also occur during pregnancy and are called *gestational diabetes.* This condition occurs in about 6 to 10 percent of all pregnancies. The mother does not have to worry about congenital malformations but still has to worry about the other problems listed previously. She also has to worry that she will develop permanent diabetes some years after the pregnancy.

Problems for the developing baby

Besides the concern for congenital malformations in the fetus exposed to high blood glucose during conception, there are more concerns for the fetus exposed to high blood glucose throughout the pregnancy. The fetus is able to make insulin, the storage hormone. In the presence of high glucose, more insulin is made and the fetus starts to store fat and become large in the shoulders, chest, abdomen, arms, and legs. These babies may weigh more than 8 and a half pounds (4 kilograms) at birth and create a very difficult delivery, often ending in a caesarean section.

If the father has diabetes but the mother does not, the baby is not in danger of any of these problems. The environment that the fetus is exposed to is responsible for the damage that occurs.

REMEMBER

All the trouble that occurs for the mother as well as the growing fetus can be prevented by very tight control of the blood glucose, starting with the time before conception of the baby and continuing right through delivery.

Screening pregnant women is vital at 24 weeks and 28 weeks of pregnancy, the time when gestational diabetes shows up. A screening test is done by feeding the mother 50 grams of glucose and measuring the blood glucose one hour after the feeding. If the glucose is less than 140 mg/dL (7.8 mmol/L), it's considered normal. If the test result is greater than 140 mg/dL, a definitive test for gestational diabetes is done.

Circumventing cognitive decline

People with established Type 2 diabetes face a higher risk of cognitive problems, including memory difficulties, slower thinking, and a greater chance of developing dementia, including Alzheimer's disease. The reasons are complex, but it's likely due to a combination of long-term damage to blood vessels in the brain, increased inflammation, and the harmful effects of consistently high blood sugar levels on brain cells themselves.

The encouraging news is that better blood glucose control through a combination of lifestyle changes and, if needed, medical treatment can help reduce the risk of cognitive decline. Keeping your diabetes well managed not only protects your heart, kidneys, and eyes, but may also help preserve your memory and thinking skills as you age.

Treating Established Diabetes

When prediabetes progresses to Type 2 diabetes, it means the body's ability to regulate blood glucose has declined further. This usually calls for closer monitoring and more structured treatment to help prevent complications such as heart disease, kidney damage, or vision loss. In addition to regular HbA1c tests, some people may benefit from continuous glucose monitoring (CGM) devices, which track glucose levels throughout the day and night. In some cases, CGMs are connected to systems that help guide or even automate medication adjustments, offering a more responsive and personalized approach to diabetes care.

Focusing on diet and lifestyle

Many people diagnosed with Type 2 diabetes, particularly in its early stages, can still achieve excellent glucose control through diet and lifestyle changes alone. Regular physical activity, balanced nutrition, weight management, and attention to sleep and stress can significantly reduce blood glucose levels. In these cases, it may be possible to maintain an HbA1c within the recommended range without needing medication, though regular follow-up remains important.

Understanding when medications are necessary

When medication is required, doctors can choose from a range of options. These include metformin (which improves insulin sensitivity), SGLT2 inhibitors (which help the kidneys excrete excess glucose), DPP-4 inhibitors (which help increase insulin release), sulfonylureas (which stimulate the pancreas to produce more insulin), and insulin itself, when needed.

Another important class is the GLP-1 receptor agonists, which work by enhancing insulin release, slowing digestion, and helping with appetite control. Some well-known GLP-1 drugs include semaglutide (Ozempic, Wegovy), liraglutide (Victoza, Saxenda), and dulaglutide (Trulicity). Originally developed for diabetes management, certain formulations of these medications have now been approved specifically for weight loss, opening new possibilities for people living with Type 2 diabetes, especially those with obesity or weight-related health risks.

Despite their recent surge in popularity with celebrities and the media, the long-term benefits or harm of these drugs (when they're used solely for weight loss in the absence of diabetes) is yet to be fully established, both in terms of their potential for side effects, and their ability to maintain weight loss for the long term. Lifestyle changes, on the other hand, to address weight loss, provide great opportunities for improvement of overall health and fitness.

TIP

For more information about diabetes and how to manage it, check out our series of *Diabetes For Dummies* books.

IN THIS CHAPTER

» **Realizing that your choices make all the difference**

» **Shopping and eating in a new way**

» **Moving your body**

» **Considering medications**

» **Weighing the pros and cons of weight loss surgery**

Chapter **4**

Stopping Prediabetes in Its Tracks

t's time to start thinking about an overall approach to reversing prediabetes and turning yourself (specifically your body) into the person you want to be. No one can make this change for you. You have to make the decision and stick to it. Doctors can offer advice, but you meet with your doctor for just a few minutes every few months. The rest of the time you are on your own.

I'm reminded of a story told about the great saxophone player John Coltrane. He was often invited by Miles Davis, a great trumpeter, to play with his band. Coltrane had one problem. When he started playing a solo, he couldn't stop. Someone asked him why his solos were so extended, and Coltrane said, "I get involved in this thing and I don't know how to stop." Davis told him, "Try taking the saxophone out of your mouth."

The point is that you do have the power to shape your life and your health. The earlier you start, the better, because some conditions become irreversible after a time. But a good decision made even after a lifetime of bad habits can have benefits. For example, cigarette smokers are subject to sudden death. Within days of stopping smoking, your risk of sudden death greatly diminishes or even disappears. Just take that cigarette out of your mouth!

In this chapter, our goal is to get you thinking about specific actions you can take that will stop the onslaught of prediabetes and put you on the path toward better health. I focus on changing your relationship with food and exercise, considering medications, and weighing the benefits and risks of weight loss surgery.

Halting and Reversing Bad Choices

Prediabetes is influenced by several choices. Some of the most important choices include:

>> The choice to eat just a little more food each day than you burn up in your daily activities, resulting in the storage of fat

>> The choice to sit passively in front of a screen instead of actively moving your body for at least a half hour each day, seven days a week

>> The choice to drink sugary soft drinks instead of water

>> The choice to eat foods that are high in saturated fats (see Chapter 5), and trans-fatty acids and low in dietary fiber

>> The choice to consume excessive salt (exceeding the daily Recommended Daily Intake, RDI, which varies from country to country), which could come from processed foods, prepared foods, or adding additional salt at the table. It's important to establish your body's own needs with a nutrition professional

>> The choice to drink alcohol

>> The choice to skip pills that lower your blood pressure and blood fats

>> The choice not to allow a health care professional to monitor you regularly for increased glucose, fats, and blood pressure

Do you recognize yourself in this list? You may even be making additional bad choices that I didn't list here, such as using illegal drugs. Whatever bad choices you are making, they are choices. You may feel that some of them are out of your control — that you are addicted to something like food or alcohol. Even then, you have the choice to seek help. Millions of people have done so and reversed their own bad choices.

Our intention is not to make you feel bad about yourself. We point out all the bad choices you are making as a way to get you to understand that you can turn those choices around into good ones. You have the power! You can take many different approaches to reversing your choices. In the sections that follow, we offer several options in the hopes that at least one will work for you.

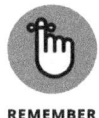

You don't have to feel out of control. You can prevent or reverse prediabetes and avoid all the short-term and long-term complications of diabetes. You can live a long, high-quality life. You just have to start by recognizing that you have a choice.

Becoming a Brand New Shopper

Making good choices begins with what you buy. Instead of the market influencing what you buy, you need your good instincts to determine what you carry out of the store. Follow these suggestions and you will not only improve your diet but also save money.

In doing your shopping, remember the old cliché: "Out of sight, out of mind." Here are some suggestions to maximize the healthy content of your shopping basket:

>> Always have a list of what you need to buy and stick with it.

>> Eat a light snack such as a piece of fruit before you go to the store so that you aren't hungry.

>> Shop at the same store each time so you know where everything is in the store.

>> Go into the store as seldom as possible.

>> Don't walk every aisle. Avoid the tempting aisles such as the bakery and the loose foods that often result in a little tasting.

>> Get into the habit of reading food nutrition labels.

>> Never take a free sample. The sample items are generally high in calories and high in price. Stores want you to buy what they profit from the most.

>> If you must bring your kids, give them a healthy snack before shopping. And firmly put their high calorie, low nutrition snack choices back on the shelf.

>> At the checkout lane, keep your eyes straight ahead and don't pick up the little goodies placed there to tempt you.

Focusing on fresh

One of the major new directions in eating healthy is focusing on fresh, local foods. Doing so makes great sense. Fresh foods are definitely the most delicious and nutritious way you can eat. If they come from local growers, they were picked at the peak of their taste — unlike so-called "fresh" foods shipped from far away, which are picked before they are ripe to give them the longest shelf time. Often those foods never fully ripen, and you never get to enjoy the real taste of the fruit or vegetable. They may not even be grown for taste but only to maintain their shape and appearance before rotting.

Another major benefit of eating fresh, local food is the ability to know the farmer. Local farmers welcome direct connections to the people who buy their produce. They may put their website on the produce so you can look up how each farmer grows their crops. Do they use sprays? Are they organic? Do they use growing methods that renew the soil?

One of the best ways to get fresh, local produce is to go to your local farmers' market. It doesn't get much better than this. You get to taste the food before you buy it — something that supermarkets are just beginning to offer. You get to talk to the farmer directly. They have often picked the crop just hours before. Plus, many different farms are usually represented at a farmers' market. You don't have to settle for one kind of corn or broccoli. The fact that you have a choice is highly motivating to the farmer to bring the best and sell for less.

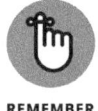

REMEMBER

Food at farmers' markets may sometimes be a little more expensive because the farmer does not use cheap ingredients in growing it. If you can afford it, pay a little more for quality. The taste will make your investment worthwhile.

Of course, the very best way to get fresh, local produce is to grow yourself.

If you don't have property on which to grow food, just grow some herbs on a counter in front of a window. The sense of satisfaction as you eat your own produce is worth every minute you spend growing it.

Reading labels like an expert

Packaged foods require labels to tell you what you are getting. How often do you actually read the label? It contains an enormous amount of useful information.

>> **How many servings are contained in the package?** One package does not necessarily mean one serving. With some food items, that fact is obvious. (A box of pasta or rice clearly contains multiple servings.) But other times, the serving size is may not be very transparent and may even be misleading. You may, for example, be drinking a soft drink from a bottle or can which seems like an individual serving, but looking at the label will reveal that it is meant for more people, and you won't realize this unless you read the label.

Be warned that food manufacturers may try to trip you up in this way and be mindful of how many calories you're actually consuming!

>> **Is there any trans fat in the food?** *Trans fat* is a form of fat that is found in foods naturally in tiny amounts but was added by food manufacturers to increase shelf life and to replace butter because trans fat is much cheaper. Trans fats, also known as trans fatty acids, partially hydrogenated oils (PHOs), or shortening, are harmful fats found in many processed foods, baked goods, margarine, and fried foods. They raise LDL ("bad") cholesterol, lower HDL ("good") cholesterol, and, even in small amounts, significantly increase the risk of heart disease, heart attacks, and strokes.

The World Health Organization (WHO) recommends limiting trans fat intake to less than 1 percent of daily energy, or under 2.2 grams per day in a 2,000-calorie diet. It urges replacing trans fats with healthier unsaturated fats and launched the REPLACE initiative to eliminate industrially produced trans fats globally. In response, many countries have introduced strict policies, including limits or full bans on added trans fats. Nations such as Denmark, Austria, Norway, Singapore, Saudi Arabia, and Thailand have successfully eliminated industrial trans fats from their food supply. As of 2025, nearly 60 countries have adopted best-practice policies, covering almost half the world's population, with efforts continuing to expand global protection.

TIP

Look for trans fats in margarines, cake mixes, dried soup mixes, baked goods such as donuts and cookies, potato chips, candies, whipped toppings, and some "healthy" breakfast cereals. Keep trans fats completely out of your diet. The naturally occurring trans fats are okay, however.

>> **How many calories are in a serving?** Calorie labelling on food can be a useful guide, especially when it highlights the high energy content of ultra-processed or poor-quality foods likely to contribute to weight gain. However, it's important to recognize the limits of calorie counts. Foods rich in natural, healthy fats such as nuts, seeds, olive oil, and avocados, may be high in calories but can actually support weight management and blood glucose regulation when eaten as part of a balanced, nutrient-dense diet. Context matters more than numbers alone.

>> **What are the levels of saturated fat and salt?** A nutrition label should provide these details. Be sure to take these figures into account when you are purchasing foods. In some countries, this is accompanied by a traffic light color guide, which makes it easier to see at a glance whether a product is high (red), medium (amber), or low (green) in saturated fat and salt. Choosing products with more green or amber indicators and fewer reds can help you manage your intake of these and support cardiovascular health and blood

pressure. However, this system is quite "broad brush," as not all saturated fats have the same health effects, for example, full-fat dairy especially in the form of yogurt or cheese has not been linked to an increased risk of cardiovascular disease and may even be protective for prediabetes and diabetes.

» **What is the sugar content?** This factor is particularly relevant when it comes to prediabetes. Sugar is usually listed on nutrition labels as "total sugars" under the "carbohydrates (of which sugars)" section, which includes both naturally occurring sugars and added sugars.

The traffic light system on the front of packaging (in countries where it's applied) uses red, amber, and green to indicate whether a product is high, medium, or low in total sugars, making it easy to see at a glance how much sugar the food contains.

» **What is on the list of ingredients?** You can find freshly baked bread with a list of 4 or 5 ingredients. Maybe there are added seeds or even vitamins and minerals. But it's also possible to buy heavily processed bread with twenty or more ingredients, which may include rapeseed oil, spirit vinegar, calcium propionate (a preservative), soya flour, emulsifiers (such as mono- and diacetyl tartaric acid esters of mono- and diglycerides of fatty acids), palm oil, along with other possible additives and conditioners that are there to add shelf life and for the convenience of the producer, not for the good of your health. While there may be no specific recommendations against the use of these additives, there is increasing concerns that some of the many ingredients you do not recognize may be having negative effects on health including for example, disrupting your gut microbiome.

» **Is it an ultra-processed food?** This question is the follow on from the last. Ultra-processed foods are industrial products made mostly from refined ingredients such as sugars, oils, starches, and synthetic additives such as flavorings, colorings, and emulsifiers, with little or no whole food content. Designed for convenience, long shelf life, and strong taste appeal, they include items such as sugary drinks, packaged snacks, processed meats, and ready meals. Typically high in calories, salt, and unhealthy fats but low in fiber and nutrients, these foods have been linked to obesity, Type 2 diabetes, cancers, heart disease, and other health risks.

The NOVA classification system, developed in Brazil, has been influential in identifying ultra-processed foods and highlighting their role in poor dietary patterns, and apps such as "YUKA" can support consumers in identifying them by analyzing and scoring foods based on phone scanning of bar code information.

Knowing what foods and ingredients to avoid at all costs

You should avoid a few "foods" altogether. We put the word "foods" in quotation marks because these items are not nutritious but just sources of *empty calories:* calories without vitamins, minerals, or fiber. When you avoid these items, you leave room for nutritious foods that promote health. Trans fats, which we discuss in the previous section, fall into this category. The other main ones include:

>> **Bleached white flour:** The bleaching process removes vitamins, minerals, and fiber, leaving empty calories. Read the food label. Look for unbleached white flour or whole wheat flour in the ingredients. Many prepared cakes and cookies contain bleached white flour. Their ingredients list often say "enriched" white flour, suggesting that vitamins and minerals have been added back, but the result is not as good as not bleaching the flour in the first place.

>> **Soft drinks with sweeteners:** A sweetened soft drink contains absolutely no nutrition. These drinks are the number one source of energy intake in the US population, but the type of energy they contain isn't what your body needs. Soft drinks contribute in a major way to the body fat that leads to prediabetes and Type 2 diabetes. You should also avoid soft drinks with artificial sweeteners. Increasing concerns that artificial sweeteners are as likely to result in weight gain as sugar, with several large-scale studies showing a positive association between artificial sweetener use and increased body weight and fat stores, particularly with long-term consumption. There are also worries about their broader impact on health, such as potential alterations to the gut microbiome, which may influence metabolism and appetite regulation, though more research is needed to fully understand these effects.

>> **High fructose corn syrup:** This very sweet and highly processed product contains little or no nutritional value. It's another so-called "food" that food manufacturers created. Corn starch is processed to yield glucose, which is further processed to yield fructose, a sugar that is sweeter than glucose. The fructose is then added back to corn syrup to produce high fructose corn syrup (HFCS). HFCS is about as sweet as sugar from sugar cane or beets but is much cheaper. It also extends the shelf life of processed foods.

TIP

Here's how to avoid HFCS:

● Limit the processed foods you eat.

● Avoid foods with added sugar or artificial sweeteners.

● Don't drink soda.

- Eat fresh fruit instead of canned fruit.
- If you eat canned fruit, buy only fruit canned in its own juices.

If you go on the Internet and look for "foods to avoid at all costs," you can come up with many other suggestions, including certain artificial sweeteners, monosodium glutamate, sugar, and palm oil.

Rethinking How You Eat

Changing your eating habits is tough. You learned those habits by watching your parents for perhaps eighteen years. You speak like your parents, you gesture like your parents, and you probably eat like your parents, so take a good look at them. Do your parents look healthy and younger than their real age? Or do they take a lot of pills for chronic diseases that you would rather avoid?

Becoming your own personal chef

If you have ever built anything, you realize that one of the great pleasures is knowing where every screw, bolt, and joint is located. The same concept is true if you cook for yourself or participate in the cooking. Just as growing your own food gives you great personal satisfaction, cooking your own food makes you feel a connection to your body and your health. What are the benefits?

>> You choose the ingredients.

>> You choose how long to cook the food.

>> You choose how much to prepare.

>> You save money compared to eating out.

TIP

If you are nervous about cooking your own food, by all means take a cooking class. You can find classes for every type of ethnic food, so if you love Italian or Chinese, you can learn all you need to know to make your favorite food regularly.

Navigating a restaurant meal when you must

If you just don't feel like cooking, or if you must be away from home, you have to learn how to eat for health at a restaurant. That's a tougher assignment than you may think. You often don't know what is in the food you are eating. You always get portions that are larger than you should eat, often twice as large. Here are some tips you need to know about the restaurant experience:

>> **No particular ethnic food is better than any other.** You can get a healthful or an unhealthful meal in any restaurant. Some restaurants, such as fast food restaurants, require more careful planning.

>> **If you choose a restaurant you can walk to and from,** you get some extra exercise that helps make up for the extra calories you may consume.

>> **You can check out most restaurants' menus online** and make sure they offer choices that are good for you.

>> **You can call ahead and ask if the chef will accommodate your needs.** For example, ask if they can:

- Reduce the fat in a dish

- Serve gravies and sauces on the side

- Bake, broil, or poach rather than fry or sauté

>> **You want to find out whether the restaurant has special meals for people with diabetes.** Those meals are fine for people with prediabetes as well.

>> **You want to drink water or eat a small snack before you go** so that you won't be driven by hunger to make bad choices.

>> **If you reduce the calories you consume during the day prior to going** to the restaurant, you allow yourself a few more calories at the restaurant.

>> **You can ask the waiter not to serve bread at your table.**

>> **If you're dining with your partner,** sharing one meal is ideal.

>> **You shouldn't even look at the dessert menu.**

REMEMBER

You are completely in control of the choices you make. You can get wonderful food at a restaurant and still stay within the boundaries of the plan you have made for yourself.

Getting your portions in check

Many times people eat without very much awareness of the quality or quantity of the food being consumed. Mindful eating, perhaps with an expression of conscious gratitude at the beginning of a meal is a powerful tool in considering and appreciating your food.

Understanding what you are eating can be easier if you keep a food diary. Don't wait until the end of the day to remember what you ate; write everything down right after eating, both the type of food and the quantity. If you wait, you may forget.

Often the food choices that the person is making are excellent. The problem is in the portions. Figure 4-1 shows the difference between the usual portions that people report they are eating at first and the appropriate portions of food.

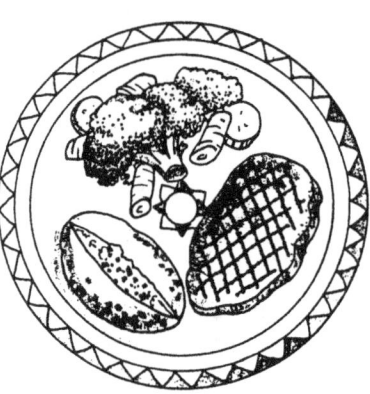 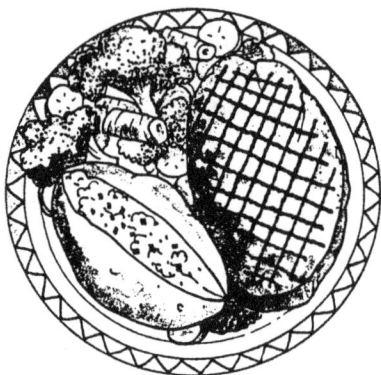

FIGURE 4-1:
The plate on the left shows the appropriate portion size. The one on the right shows what many people eat.

You can see the difference. The larger steak has more than 600 kilocalories compared to the 220 kilocalories of the smaller steak. A modern bagel has 350 kilocalories compared to the 140 kilocalories of a bagel twenty years ago. An order of French fries now has 610 kilocalories compared to 210 kilocalories twenty years ago. Even modern coffee has sweeteners that bring a cup up to 350 kilocalories compared with 45 kilocalories twenty years ago. Is it any wonder that people are putting on more weight?

Reducing portion size can be key to improving health. What a simple and amazing approach to weight loss! You don't have to give up the foods you love, just eat half as much of each.

TIP

While you're at it, take more time to enjoy your meals. Slow down the pace of your eating. You allow yourself more time to enjoy your partner and your family, and you feel full at a much lower level of food. Slowing down the pace of eating gives your brain more time to recognize that you have eaten enough.

REMEMBER

Portion size and reducing calorie intake is important for achieving and maintaining a healthy weight, but the foods we eat and their nutritional value in a healthy diet like the Mediterranean diet is also important. We discuss this is in later chapters of this book.

Putting Your Body in Gear

Exercise is an absolutely essential element to preventing and managing prediabetes. Regular physical activity helps the body use insulin more efficiently, lowers blood glucose levels, and supports weight management, all of which are key in reducing the risk of progression to Type 2 diabetes. Even moderate activities such as brisk walking, cycling, or swimming can make a significant difference when done consistently.

Embracing exercise

Are you afraid of exercise? You shouldn't be. No one says you have to wear spandex and put yourself front-and-center in an exercise class this very minute. You have lots of options close to home that enable you to get moving in a way that's comfortable to you. You will soon begin to enjoy the "buzz," perhaps with the added pleasure of exercising in company and in nature.

What you should really fear is *not* exercising, because your body absolutely requires it. The Romans had it right: "A sound mind in a sound body." If you are older than forty and haven't exercised in recent years, you should see your physician and get their agreement that you can exercise. They may tell you how vigorously to exercise or leave it to you to decide.

As you exercise more and more vigorously, the benefits increase dramatically. You will probably lose weight. Your mental state will improve. Other people will start telling you how well you look. And at some point, you will feel a chemical high when you really exercise vigorously. That is when you are getting the most benefit, physically and psychologically.

Getting a walking start

Walking offers a wide range of health benefits, making it one of the simplest and most accessible forms of exercise. It helps improve cardiovascular health, supports weight management, reduces blood sugar levels, and boosts mood and mental well-being. Tracking your steps using a pedometer, smartphone, or fitness tracker can be a motivating way to set and achieve daily activity goals, with many people aiming for 7,000 to 10,000 steps a day as a practical target.

Beyond the physical benefits, walking can easily become an enjoyable pastime. Exploring local parks, walking with friends or family, listening to music or podcasts, or simply enjoying the sights and sounds of nature can make walking something to look forward to each day. This combination of health benefits and enjoyment makes walking an excellent habit for long-term well-being.

Adding Medications to Your Daily Routine

Lifestyle changes such as improved diet, increased physical activity, and weight loss remain the gold standard for managing prediabetes, some doctors prescribe medications such as metformin to help reduce the risk of progression to Type 2 diabetes. When metformin is used for prediabetes, it is often prescribed "off license" or "off label," meaning it is being used for a purpose not officially approved by medicines regulatory agencies, though there is evidence to support its effectiveness.

Multiple large studies have shown that metformin can significantly lower the risk of developing Type 2 diabetes in people with prediabetes, with risk reductions ranging from 31 to 42 percent compared to control groups. However, these same studies consistently demonstrate that intensive lifestyle interventions are even more effective than medication, with reductions in diabetes risk of up to 58 percent, and without the potential side effects associated with drug therapy. Lifestyle changes also have broader health benefits, such as improving cardiovascular health and overall well-being, making them the preferred first-line approach for most people with prediabetes.

The rise of weight managing medications

In recent years, new injectable weight loss medications, such as GLP-1 receptor agonists including semaglutide (Ozempic, Wegovy) and liraglutide (Victoza, Saxenda), have introduced new opportunities for the treatment of obesity and prediabetes as well as diabetes prevention. These drugs work by mimicking hormones that regulate appetite and blood sugar, leading to significant weight loss and improved glucose control in people at risk of diabetes. Early evidence suggests that these medications can help lower blood sugar and may reduce the risk of progression from prediabetes to Type 2 diabetes at least in the short term, particularly in people who are overweight or obese. See Chapter 3 for more information on these drugs.

Weighing in on the risks of medications

Despite the promise of medications such as metformin and newer weight loss drugs, there are important limitations and unknowns to consider. Side effects such as gastrointestinal discomfort, nausea, and, rarely, more serious complications can occur with both metformin and GLP-1 receptor agonists. The long-term safety of newer injectable medications is still being evaluated, and it is not yet clear how sustained use may affect health over many years.

It's important also to remember that medications may not address the underlying lifestyle factors that contribute to prediabetes and may not provide the same broad health benefits as diet and exercise for CVD prevention and beyond. For these reasons, experts generally recommend that medications be considered only when lifestyle interventions are not enough, and always as part of a comprehensive approach to diabetes prevention. The next few years are likely to reveal more "real world" experience and evidence of the potential benefits and harms of these medications.

Tackling Prediabetes through Surgery

You may think that surgery should be a last resort in the management of prediabetes and the prevention of — and many experts would agree. While bariatric (weight loss) surgery has shown quite dramatic and consistent benefits for people with established Type 2 diabetes, the evidence for its use specifically in prediabetes is much less convincing. Most large studies and reviews, such as the one published in the *American Journal of Medicine* in March 2009, focus on people who already have Type 2 diabetes, showing high rates of improvement or remission and substantial weight loss. However, you find far less research on the long-term outcomes and risks of surgery in people with prediabetes, and it is not clear that the benefits outweigh the risks for this group — especially considering that prediabetes can often be reversed through lifestyle changes without the need for invasive procedures.

For people with severe or morbid obesity (typically defined as a body mass index (BMI) over 40, or over 35 with significant health problems), surgery may be considered if other treatment options have failed, particularly if there is a strong family history of diabetes or other major risk factors. However, surgery carries its own risks and potential complications, and the long-term effects for people with prediabetes are still not fully understood. For most individuals with prediabetes, focusing on lifestyle interventions such as improving diet, increasing physical activity, and achieving modest weight loss remains the safest and most effective first-line approach.

Some of the major benefits of *bariatric surgery* (surgery for obesity) are:

>> Significant weight loss

>> Normalization of blood glucose

>> Normalization of blood pressure

>> Normalization of high cholesterol

>> Improvement in heart disease

>> Improvement in lung disease

>> Improvement in *sleep apnea* (a condition characterized by episodes of not breathing while you're sleeping)

>> Improvement in asthma

>> Improvement in regurgitation of stomach contents

>> Improvement in urinary stress incontinence

>> Improvement in low back pain

>> Improvement in quality of life

That's a long list. But bariatric surgery is not all positive. You must take the risks and complications into account. The decision you make must weigh the benefits against those risks and complications, which include:

>> Death, which occurs in 1 in 300 surgeries in a good surgical center and is due to the heart disease associated with the obesity.

>> *Pulmonary embolism* — the formation of a clot in the legs that breaks off and goes into the lungs. Sudden shortness of breath and chest pain result.

>> Gastrointestinal tract leak from the surgery where the intestines are stapled. A severe abdominal infection can result.

>> Bowel obstruction when scar tissue forms.

>> Stricture where scar tissue blocks the intestine.

>> Gallstones with pain under the right ribs.

>> Infections such as pneumonia or abscess in the abdomen.

>> Nutritional deficiencies such as protein deficiency, vitamin deficiency, or mineral deficiency.

>> Excessive weight loss.

None of these risks or complications of surgery (with the exception of the first one, obviously) are irreversible or permanent. And to put the risks in perspective, keep in mind that the purpose of the surgery is to prevent eventual blindness, kidney failure, nerve disease, or heart disease.

Two standard operations are now most commonly performed for weight loss: gastric bypass and sleeve gastrectomy. In each case, the word gastric refers to the stomach.

Gastric bypass

In this surgery, the stomach is divided into a small upper pouch and a large lower pouch. In addition, the small intestine is divided near where it meets the large intestine. The lower part of the small intestine is attached to the small upper stomach pouch. The large lower pouch of the stomach empties into the rest of the small intestine, which is reconnected to the lower small intestine near where it joins the large intestine. The small upper pouch of the stomach makes it impossible to eat much food at a meal, and the short length of the small intestine before it enters the large intestine significantly decreases absorption of food.

This operation results in the greatest loss of weight but also the most frequent occurrence of vitamin and mineral deficiencies. Patients who have this surgery typically lose 60 to 70 percent of their excess weight.

Sleeve gastrectomy

This is now the most commonly performed weight loss surgery. In this procedure, a large portion of the stomach is removed, leaving a narrow "sleeve." This restricts the amount of food that can be eaten but does not affect absorption. Patients typically lose 50 to 60 percent of their excess body weight, and the risk of vitamin and mineral deficiencies is lower than with gastric bypass.

Gastric banding, once common, is now rarely performed due to lower long-term effectiveness and higher complication rates compared to these two procedures.

2
Getting
a Diagnosis

Chapter **5**

Spotting the Metabolic Syndrome

I f you read some or all the chapters that have come before this one, you know that we talk a lot about the importance of a healthy lifestyle. So far, our focus has been solely on getting healthy in order to prevent or reverse prediabetes. In this chapter, we turn your attention to another condition that may develop as a result of an unhealthy lifestyle: the metabolic syndrome. The metabolic syndrome has had many other names: *metabolic syndrome X, syndrome X, insulin resistance syndrome,* and *CHAOS.* Nowadays these terms have largely been replaced with the convention of simply using the term metabolic syndrome. Metabolic syndrome is a cluster of conditions, including elevated blood pressure, high blood sugar, excess abdominal fat, and abnormal cholesterol or triglyceride levels that occur together and significantly increase the risk of heart disease, Type 2 diabetes, and stroke.

Why are we bringing up this condition in a book about prediabetes? Two reasons:

» The two conditions have a great deal in common. Their causes are similar, and the threats they pose to your body are equally severe.

>> You combat the metabolic syndrome just as you do prediabetes: by changing your eating habits, getting more exercise, and taking other steps to improve your lifestyle.

So, if you're concerned about prediabetes, chances are you need to be concerned about the metabolic syndrome as well. And if you're willing to take the necessary steps to halt and reverse prediabetes, you'll get twice the bang for your buck because you'll be combating the metabolic syndrome at the same time.

In this chapter, we explain exactly what the metabolic syndrome is, how to determine if you're at risk, what lab tests are done to achieve a diagnosis, and what steps to take to get back to good health. Not bad for just twelve pages!

Defining the Metabolic Syndrome

Like prediabetes, the metabolic syndrome is a condition that is often associated with *visceral* obesity, which means obesity that involves carrying your extra weight around your waistline (as opposed to in your hips and thighs, for example). If you have an apple-shaped body type, chances are you've got too much visceral fat.

However, just to keep life interesting, you don't have to be overweight to be diagnosed with the metabolic syndrome. If you have other risk factors and develop the signs and symptoms of the condition (which we describe in this chapter), you need to see your doctor even if you're thin.

As early as 1947, patients who showed signs of the metabolic syndrome were described by a French physician. This doctor made the connection between upper body obesity and diabetes, coronary heart disease, high cholesterol, and gout.

But only in 1988 did Dr. Gerald Reaven propose (in a lecture to the American Diabetes Association) that insulin resistance is the underlying cause of the metabolic syndrome. As we explain in Chapter 2, *insulin resistance* occurs when the insulin in your body stops working effectively.

The metabolic syndrome shares a lot of the features of prediabetes and responds to similar treatment. Having the metabolic syndrome can also predispose you to developing diabetes. Recent estimates suggest that around one in three US adults, approximately 34 percent, has metabolic syndrome, according to data from the

National Health and Nutrition Examination Survey (NHANES) published by the Centers for Disease Control and Prevention (CDC). Left untreated, this condition can lead to a fate similar to that of diabetes: a fatal heart attack.

Research suggests that the metabolic syndrome is also associated with higher rates of cancer and worse outcomes for cancers of the breast, prostate, large intestine, and other organs. Excess insulin may stimulate the growth of tumors.

Metabolic syndrome and inflammation

High blood glucose is a central feature of metabolic syndrome and plays a key role in triggering low-grade systemic inflammation, a persistent, mild activation of the immune system that can quietly damage tissues over time. Even when blood sugar levels are only moderately elevated, they can disrupt normal cellular processes and stimulate the production of inflammatory molecules such as C-reactive protein (CRP) and interleukin-6 (IL-6). A major driver of this response is oxidative stress — an imbalance between the production of harmful molecules known as free radicals and the body's ability to neutralize them with antioxidants. Elevated glucose levels can increase oxidative stress within cells, leading to cellular damage and further inflammation.

This combination of oxidative stress and low-grade inflammation creates a harmful internal environment that underlies many chronic diseases. It contributes to the development and progression of atherosclerosis and cardiovascular disease, Type 2 diabetes, non-alcoholic fatty liver disease, and even some neurodegenerative conditions and cancers. Inflammation itself worsens insulin resistance, creating a vicious cycle in which poor glucose control fuels inflammation, which in turn leads to even higher blood sugar levels. Recognizing the interconnected roles of high blood glucose, oxidative stress, and inflammation is crucial to understanding how metabolic syndrome evolves and why it poses such a significant long-term threat to health.

Determining Your Level of Risk

In this section, we explain who is most at risk for the metabolic syndrome. Having a single risk factor is not something to panic about. However, if you recognize yourself in several of the descriptions that follow, you definitely want to schedule a chat with your doctor about this condition.

Having a genetic predisposition

Most studies of the metabolic syndrome indicate that there is a hereditary component. Here are two key reasons for this conclusion:

>> The metabolic syndrome tends to cluster in families.

>> When *identical twins* (twins from a single egg) are compared with *nonidentical twins* (twins from two different eggs) for the development of the features of the metabolic syndrome, the identical twins have common features of the metabolic syndrome much more often.

However, identical twins do not *always* match up for the development of the metabolic syndrome. In other words, one twin in the set may develop the metabolic syndrome, and the other may not. This fact suggests that lifestyle and environment also play a part in developing the condition.

Getting older

As people get older, the incidence of the metabolic syndrome increases greatly. In the US, nearly half of adults over age 60 are affected, according to data from the CDC.

Unfortunately, you can't do anything about aging (just as you can't do anything about your genetic heritage). Fortunately, you *can* take action in response to the remaining risk factors. Keep reading to find out how.

Gaining weight

As you gain visceral fat (the kind that accumulates around your belly), your body's insulin becomes less effective. Your pancreas has to pump out more insulin to get energy into your muscles. This loss of insulin effectiveness is called *insulin resistance.* As you push more glucose into your cells, you are also creating more fat, and you gain more weight. The result is a further increase in insulin resistance. At some point your insulin can no longer keep up, and your blood glucose rises into the diabetic range.

Here's the kicker: You may develop the metabolic syndrome even if your weight is completely normal!

Slim people who have the metabolic syndrome were previously said to be *metabolically obese.* The phrase implies that even though their weight is in the normal range, their metabolism (the process of turning food into energy) is similar to that of an overweight person.

The term "metabolically obese" is still used informally, but more precise terms are preferred now, such as "MONW" (Metabolically Obese Normal Weight) or "TOFI" (Thin Outside, Fat Inside). Also less emphasis today is on BMI alone, and more on waist circumference and body composition to discern between healthy muscle or bone density contributing to an increased weight as opposed to fat.

REMEMBER

Even people with a normal weight (as measured by BMI) can develop metabolic syndrome if they have excess visceral fat or other risk factors — a profile sometimes called "metabolically unhealthy normal weight."

TIP

If your BMI is toward the high end of normal, and if you recognize that you have signs and symptoms of the metabolic syndrome (which I describe in the next section), you need to lower your weight further.

Living a sedentary lifestyle

Another major factor in developing the metabolic syndrome is living an unhealthy lifestyle. If you don't get much physical activity and you consume excess calories, you are living a lifestyle that promotes the metabolic syndrome. Often referred to as a *sedentary lifestyle*, it is strongly associated with the signs and symptoms of the metabolic syndrome.

Here's the great news: You can take control of this risk factor. When people with the metabolic syndrome follow an exercise program for 20 weeks, up to 30 percent of them no longer have signs or symptoms of the metabolic syndrome!

HOW INSULIN RESISTANCE DEVELOPS

As visceral fat accumulates, it acts differently than *subcutaneous* fat (fat that is located between your skin and the wall of your abdomen, arms, legs, and chest). Insulin usually causes fat storage, but visceral fat resists that action and releases large amounts of substances called *free fatty acids.* These excessive free fatty acids in the blood cause resistance to insulin in the liver and muscles, with these results:

- The production of new glucose is stimulated in the liver.

- The muscles take in a reduced amount of glucose from the blood.

(continued)

(continued)

As fat cells become filled, they resist the storage of additional fat, and it starts to be stored in your muscles, liver, and pancreas, further increasing insulin resistance in those organs.

Another substance produced by visceral fat is an enzyme that causes the production of more cortisol. Visceral fat may influence hormone levels, including cortisol, which can further promote fat accumulation and insulin resistance — creating a self-reinforcing cycle.

Becoming aware of other risk factors

Several other factors increase your odds of developing the metabolic syndrome. Some are irreversible, but others are within your control:

» **Postmenopausal status:** The hormones that are secreted while a woman has periods may protect against the development of the metabolic syndrome and explain why cardiovascular disease occurs so much later in females than in males.

» **Tobacco exposure:** Smoking greatly increases the risk for the metabolic syndrome. Unfortunately, exposure to second-hand smoke does as well.

» **Low socioeconomic status:** Studies of many communities have shown that as socioeconomic status declines, the prevalence of the metabolic syndrome increases. This connection may result from unhealthy food choices and the increased stress associated with low socioeconomic status.

» **High carbohydrate diet:** People who eat lots of carbohydrates, especially *refined* (processed) carbohydrates, tend to have a higher prevalence of the metabolic syndrome. Refined carbohydrates tend to raise your glucose, insulin, and triglyceride levels while lowering your HDL (good) cholesterol. Eating more carbohydrates with low glycemic indexes (which we explain in Chapter 5) can help protect you against the metabolic syndrome.

» **Mexican-American ethnicity:** The risk of metabolic syndrome varies by ethnic group. For example, Mexican Americans, particularly women, have a higher prevalence. Other groups, such as South Asians and Native Americans, may also be at increased risk, sometimes even at lower body weights.

Recognizing Major Signs and Symptoms

Patients with the metabolic syndrome have a large number of abnormalities, many of which predispose them to heart disease and heart attacks. These abnormalities can be divided into physical signs and symptoms and laboratory abnormalities.

The metabolic syndrome has been defined by several different groups, including The National Cholesterol Education Program and the World Health Organization.

The most widely used definition of metabolic syndrome comes from a 2009 joint statement by several major health organizations. It defines metabolic syndrome as the presence of any three of the following five criteria:

>> Central obesity, defined as a waist circumference of 40 inches (102 cm) or more in men and 35 inches (88 cm) or more in women. (**Note:** Ethnicity-specific thresholds may apply; for example, lower cutoffs are recommended for people of South or East Asian descent.)

>> Elevated triglycerides, defined as 150 mg/dL (1.7 mmol/L) or higher, or being on medication to treat high triglycerides.

>> Low HDL ("good") cholesterol, defined as less than 40 mg/dL (1.0 mmol/L) in men and less than 50 mg/dL (1.3 mmol/L) in women, or being on medication to raise HDL levels.

>> Elevated blood pressure, defined as 130/85 mm Hg or higher, or taking medication for hypertension.

>> Elevated fasting blood glucose, defined as 100 mg/dL (5.6 mmol/L) or higher, or being on medication to treat elevated blood sugar.

Identifying physical signs and symptoms

The physical signs and symptoms of the metabolic syndrome often overlap with those of prediabetes. They include:

>> **High blood pressure:** This symptom may result from the increased levels of insulin in the body, which are necessary to keep the blood glucose normal.

>> **Increased abdominal visceral fat:** The waist is greater than 40 inches in men and 35 inches in women.

>> **Obesity:** Many, but not all, people with the metabolic syndrome are obese.

- **Sedentary lifestyle:** However, an active lifestyle does not rule out the metabolic syndrome.

- **Polycystic ovarian syndrome:** This group of abnormalities includes menstrual irregularity, infertility, and excess facial and body hair in females that is related to insulin resistance.

- **Cognition disorders and Alzheimer's disease:** Emerging research suggests that insulin resistance may also affect brain health and has been linked to an increased risk of cognitive decline and Alzheimer's disease. However, this connection is still being actively studied.

Looking at laboratory abnormalities

People with the metabolic syndrome have a large number of laboratory abnormalities, in addition to those that are part of the definition of the syndrome. These abnormalities contribute to the heart disease that is the outcome of untreated metabolic syndrome. Most of the abnormalities reverse with appropriate treatment.

In addition to the key lab markers used to diagnose metabolic syndrome, several other abnormalities may show up in your test results. These can indicate how your body is handling inflammation, liver health, and blood sugar regulation:

- High fasting insulin levels may point to insulin resistance, although this is not routinely tested.

- C-reactive protein (CRP) is a marker of inflammation that may be elevated in people with visceral fat and insulin resistance.

- Microalbuminuria (a small amount of protein in the urine) may indicate early kidney changes and increased cardiovascular risk.

- Nonalcoholic fatty liver disease (NAFLD) is now considered a common consequence of metabolic syndrome and may be detected through abnormal liver enzymes or imaging tests.

Reversing the Causes of the Metabolic Syndrome

Now that you understand what causes the metabolic syndrome and what it looks like, the good news is that you can take action to reverse it — and at the same time, reduce your risk of prediabetes and heart disease.

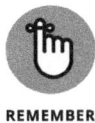

The more consistently you adopt healthy habits, the more likely you are to prevent serious complications such as heart disease and Type 2 diabetes. Examples of healthy habits include:

>> **Lose weight:** If one or both of your parents have the metabolic syndrome, do whatever you can to avoid having a body mass index of 25 or greater. Aim to keep your body weight within the healthy BMI range (18.5–24.9), and if you're at the higher end of that range and have other risk factors, even modest weight loss can help lower your blood pressure, blood sugar, and triglyceride levels.

TIP

If you are at risk for the metabolic syndrome and you have children, take action now to make sure they are never overweight!

>> **Get active:** Start walking for at least 30 minutes daily, and preferably for an hour. Make the time (see Chapter 7 for pointers). And do little diversions throughout your day to increase your activity level:

- Leave your car at home whenever possible.

- Park your car blocks from your destination so you're forced to walk the remaining distance. (You may find it easier to locate a parking space this way, which will also lower your stress level!)

- Walk up stairs instead of taking the elevator.

- Wear a pedometer and keep a record of the number of steps you walk each day. Try to add a few hundred steps whenever possible.

- Take a walk during your lunch break.

>> **Stop smoking:** I know it's easy to say and hard to do, but you simply must do it. And you also must demand that nobody smoke in your environment. Second-hand smoke greatly increases the risk for the metabolic syndrome. Consider smoking cessation programs or support tools, such as apps, counselling, or medications.

>> **Eat fewer refined carbohydrates:** Focus on reducing refined or processed carbohydrates — such as white bread, pastries, and sugary snacks. Instead, choose whole-grain, fiber-rich carbohydrates with a low glycemic index, which help stabilize blood sugar and reduce metabolic risk.

>> **Skip the sugary and diet sodas:** Choose water or unsweetened drinks over sugary beverages. Cutting back on added sugars in drinks — even those that are artificially sweetened — can support better metabolic health.

>> **Follow the Mediterranean diet or the Dietary Approaches to Stop Hypertension (DASH) diet:** The DASH diet, which was developed to treat high blood pressure, has also shown to be valuable in the metabolic syndrome. Following the DASH diet, which involves increasing your intake of fruits and vegetables, results in higher HDL cholesterol, lower triglycerides, lower blood pressure, reduced weight, and lower blood glucose. The Mediterranean diet is similar in many respects and has the added benefit of evidence for prevention of numerous chronic diseases.

Dealing with Uncontrolled Metabolic Syndrome

If you haven't been able to prevent the metabolic syndrome, you can at least minimize the damage by treating some of the consequences.

Reversing high blood glucose

Metformin is the most widely studied and commonly prescribed medication for lowering blood glucose in Type 2 diabetes, and it is also sometimes used to help prevent diabetes in people at high risk. It's important to note that although there is evidence supporting its benefit in people with metabolic syndrome to lower blood sugar and reduce the progression to diabetes, metformin is not specifically licensed (approved) for treating metabolic syndrome itself in many countries. Its use in this context is considered "off license" or "off label," meaning it's prescribed based on the doctor's judgment of benefit, but outside the formal approved indications.

As well as metformin, newer classes of medications have become available, notably the GLP-1 receptor agonists, examples include liraglutide and semaglutide. These drugs work by mimicking a natural gut hormone that stimulates insulin secretion, suppresses appetite, and can lead to weight loss. While GLP-1 agonists are approved for the treatment of Type 2 diabetes and obesity, research has shown they can improve insulin resistance and reduce blood glucose in people who have the metabolic syndrome, particularly among those who are overweight or have polycystic ovary syndrome (PCOS). Clinical trials support their beneficial effects on insulin sensitivity, fasting glucose, and body weight in these populations but their use for metabolic syndrome specifically, outside diagnosed diabetes or obesity, is still an area of ongoing research, and they are not yet routinely licensed for this broader indication.

Bariatric surgery may also be considered in obese patients with metabolic syndrome. Glucose levels can be significantly reduced and insulin resistance improvements are often seen following bariatric surgery.

Lowering your blood pressure

Numerous medications are available that can lower your blood pressure, but experts recommend a drug from the class called *Angiotensin-Converting Enzyme (ACE) inhibitors* that have shown to be especially protective of the kidneys while they lower the blood pressure. If this medication is not effective alone, your doctor may recommend adding a diuretic, which causes water loss.

Improving your blood fats (lipids)

Many drugs may be helpful here as well. Statins are amongst the most commonly prescribed medications. You can find more information in *Managing Cholesterol For Dummies* (Wiley 2025).

REMEMBER

After you have the metabolic syndrome, you can take many steps to combat it. But as with every other disease, an ounce of prevention is worth a pound of cure. Don't let yourself get to the stage where you need these medications or even surgery.

As we note earlier in the chapter, growing evidence indicates that insulin resistance, the basis for the metabolic syndrome, may play a major role in Alzheimer's disease. Making lifestyle changes now, which can slow down or reverse the metabolic syndrome and prediabetes, may do the same for Alzheimer's disease. What are you waiting for?

IN THIS CHAPTER

» Keeping an eye on your blood glucose

» Checking up on your cholesterol

» Getting acquainted with your blood pressure

» Testing for inflammation

» Figuring out if you're missing nutrients

Chapter **6**

The Testing Spectrum: Having Essential Tests and Interpreting Results

To figure out if you have prediabetes, or to figure out whether you're getting it under control after you are diagnosed, you need to be prepared to have a few essential lab tests, all of which we cover in this chapter.

And honestly, some of the most important numbers you need to know don't require any blood work at all. Instead, they're basic measurements such as height, weight, waist circumference, and blood pressure. With the exception of blood pressure, we don't discuss these measurements in this chapter. But that's not a commentary on their importance — just a vote of confidence in your ability to wield a tape measure and a bathroom scale.

Checking Your Blood Glucose Level

Blood glucose levels naturally fluctuate throughout the day in response to meals, activity, stress, and even sleep. In healthy adults, fasting blood glucose typically ranges between 70 and 100 mg/dl (3.9–5.6 mmol/L), with levels rising temporarily after eating, often up to around 140 mg/dl (7.8 mmol/L), before returning to baseline within a few hours. These variations are tightly controlled by a complex interplay of hormones, chiefly insulin and glucagon, which ensure that cells receive the energy they need while preventing blood sugar from rising too high or falling too low.

For many years, fasting blood glucose and the glucose tolerance test (GTT) discussed in Chapter 1 were the standard tools doctors used to diagnose diabetes and prediabetes. However, these tests require fasting, can be inconvenient, and are subject to day-to-day variability due to factors such as recent meals, stress, or illness. Today, the HbA1c (glycated hemoglobin) test has largely replaced these methods for routine screening and diagnosis. HbA1c reflects your average blood glucose over the past two to three months, offering a more stable and practical snapshot of your metabolic health. While HbA1c has some limitations, such as being less reliable in people with certain blood disorders, it is now the preferred test in most cases. In this chapter, we explain in detail how HbA1c works, what your results mean, and why this shift in testing matters for your health.

An emerging but still experimental approach to personal glucose tracking involves the use of continuous glucose monitors (CGMs). These wearable devices measure glucose levels in real time throughout the day and night, giving users a detailed view of how their bodies respond to food, exercise, sleep, and stress. While CGMs are primarily designed for people with diabetes, some companies now market them to people without diabetes who want to monitor their glucose for wellness or performance reasons. This includes interest from people with prediabetes who are looking for more personalized insights into their lifestyle.

TIP

CGMs are not currently recommended as a standard tool for diagnosing or managing prediabetes. Their use in this context is still under investigation, and more research is needed to confirm their value in routine preventive care.

Tracking Your Glucose for the Last 90 Days

Single tests of your blood glucose are very useful to know what's happening at any given second. But what about the other 86,399 seconds in a day? Your blood glucose can vary greatly in a few minutes, especially after you've eaten or exercised. What you need is a test that can tell you how your blood glucose has been doing for a significant length of time. The *hemoglobin A1c* (HbA1c) is that test.

Hemoglobin, the protein in red blood cells that carries oxygen, can become "glycated" when exposed to glucose in your bloodstream. The more glucose you have over time, the more glycated hemoglobin forms. The HbA1c test measures this glycation, giving an estimate of your average blood glucose over the past two to three months.

Glucose is measured in different units around the world: mg/dL (milligrams per deciliter) is common in the United States, while mmol/L (millimoles per liter) is standard in the UK, Europe, Australia, and many other countries. Similarly, HbA1c results are reported either as a percentage (%) or in mmol/mol — the latter is now the standard in most countries outside the US.

Here's what your HbA1c result means:

>> Below 42 mmol/mol (6.0 percent): This level is considered normal.

>> 42–47 mmol/mol (6.0–6.4 percent): This range is the prediabetes range. If your result is here, your average glucose is higher than normal, but not yet high enough for a diabetes diagnosis.

>> 48 mmol/mol (6.5 percent) or above: This level is the threshold for diagnosing diabetes. At this level, your average blood glucose is consistently too high.

To help you relate your HbA1c to daily glucose readings, here are some examples:

>> An HbA1c of 42 mmol/mol (6.0 percent) corresponds to an estimated average glucose (eAG) of 126 mg/dL (7.0 mmol/L).

>> An HbA1c of 48 mmol/mol (6.5 percent) corresponds to 140 mg/dL (7.8 mmol/L).

>> An HbA1c of 53 mmol/mol (7.0 percent) corresponds to 154 mg/dL (8.6 mmol/L).

These conversions show how your long-term HbA1c result relates to the glucose numbers you may see on a home monitor.

TIP

If you have prediabetes (HbA1c 42–47 mmol/mol or 6.0–6.4 percent), lifestyle changes can often help bring your levels back into the normal range. If your HbA1c reaches 48 mmol/mol (6.5 percent) or higher, this signals diabetes, and you should discuss next steps with your healthcare team.

REMEMBER

HbA1c may not be accurate in people with certain blood disorders, anemia, kidney disease, or liver disease. Also, while HbA1c is now the standard test for diagnosing diabetes and prediabetes in most countries, your doctor may recommend other tests if you have conditions that affect HbA1c reliability.

Knowing Your Cholesterol Levels

Abnormal cholesterol levels, especially high LDL ("bad") cholesterol, low HDL ("good") cholesterol, and elevated triglycerides, significantly increase the risk of heart disease in people with prediabetes, diabetes, and metabolic syndrome. *Atherosclerosis* (the build-up of fatty plaques in the walls of arteries) is the underlying cause of most cardiovascular diseases. This process begins when the inner lining of blood vessels becomes damaged, allowing cholesterol, fats, and other substances to accumulate and form plaques. Over time, these plaques can become inflamed, further damaging the artery walls and narrowing the passage for blood flow, which may eventually lead to heart attacks, strokes, or other serious complications.

Atherosclerosis develops through a combination of factors. High blood glucose from diabetes or prediabetes can directly injure blood vessel walls. High blood pressure adds mechanical stress, causing further damage. *Oxidized cholesterol* (cholesterol molecules that have been chemically altered by reactive substances in the body) is especially harmful because it triggers inflammation within the artery wall. Toxins from cigarette smoke and environmental pollutants also contribute by promoting inflammation and oxidative stress. Together, these factors create a perfect storm for plaque formation and cardiovascular disease, which is why considering these other factors is so important if you are diagnosed with prediabetes.

Simply knowing your total cholesterol isn't enough; it's essential to understand the breakdown between HDL, LDL, and triglycerides, as each plays a distinct role in cardiovascular health.

Because cholesterol isn't soluble in blood, it travels in particles called lipoproteins. There are four main types:

>> **Chylomicrons** are large particles that carry dietary fats from the intestine. They are cleared quickly from the blood and do not directly cause atherosclerosis.

>> **VLDL** (very low-density lipoprotein) particles transport triglycerides. While not as directly harmful as LDL, high levels — especially when HDL is low — can contribute to cardiovascular risk.

>> **HDL** (high-density lipoprotein) is considered "good" cholesterol because it helps remove cholesterol from the arteries.

>> **LDL** (low-density lipoprotein) is known as "bad" cholesterol because it delivers cholesterol to tissues, including artery walls, where it can contribute to plaque buildup and heart disease.

If you are being treated for abnormal blood fats, your doctor should check a fasting lipid panel (measuring total cholesterol, HDL, LDL, and triglycerides) at least once a year, or more often if needed. In some cases, non-HDL cholesterol (total cholesterol minus HDL) is also measured, especially if triglycerides are high.

Current treatment targets are more aggressive than in the past, particularly for people with diabetes or existing heart disease. For those at highest risk, guidelines recommend LDL cholesterol below 70 mg/dL (1.8 mmol/L), with even lower targets considered in some cases. HDL cholesterol above 40 mg/dL (men) or 50 mg/dL (women) is desirable, but raising HDL with medication has not been shown to reduce heart attacks. Triglycerides should be kept below 150 mg/dL (1.7 mmol/L).

If lifestyle changes aren't enough, statins are the first-line medication. If targets aren't met, ezetimibe or PCSK9 inhibitors may be added. Newer diabetes medications, such as GLP-1 receptor agonists and SGLT2 inhibitors, can also reduce cardiovascular risk, independent of their effects on cholesterol.

In metabolic syndrome, the combination of low HDL and high triglycerides is a hallmark. Treatment focuses on lifestyle changes and managing each risk factor. While the total cholesterol/HDL ratio can be a simple risk marker, the main focus is on achieving optimal LDL and non-HDL cholesterol levels.

Regular monitoring and individualized treatment are key to reducing your risk of heart disease if you have prediabetes, diabetes, or metabolic syndrome.

Deciding whether treatment is necessary

The decision to treat abnormal blood fats — dyslipidemia — is based not just on your cholesterol and triglyceride levels, but on your overall risk of having a heart attack, stroke, or other cardiovascular event. Modern guidelines use risk calculators such as SCORE2 in Europe, PREVENT in the US, or QRISK3 in the UK to estimate your 10-year (and sometimes 30-year) risk, rather than relying on simple checklists of risk factors. These calculators consider age, sex, smoking status, blood pressure, cholesterol (total, HDL, and non-HDL), diabetes, kidney function, body mass index (BMI), and sometimes family history.

Three Levels of Risk are:

>> **Highest risk (secondary prevention):** You already have established cardiovascular disease — such as a previous heart attack, stroke, or peripheral artery disease. In this group, intensive lipid-lowering therapy is nearly always recommended, regardless of your cholesterol numbers.

>> **High risk (primary prevention):** You do not have known cardiovascular disease, but your calculated risk (using a validated calculator) is above a certain threshold — often 10 percent or higher over 10 years in the UK and Europe. This group may also include people with diabetes, chronic kidney disease, or very high LDL cholesterol. Lifestyle changes and statin therapy are usually recommended.

>> **Low to moderate risk:** Your calculated risk is below the treatment threshold. Here, lifestyle modification is emphasized, and medication is generally not recommended unless other factors (such as very high LDL or strong family history) are present.

Family history, smoking, high blood pressure, low HDL, and elevated BMI are still important, but they are now integrated into risk calculators rather than used as standalone criteria. For example, the PREVENT and SCORE2 calculators incorporate these factors, along with cholesterol, blood pressure, diabetes, and kidney function, to provide a personalized risk estimate.

Current guidelines no longer use fixed LDL cholesterol cutoffs to decide when to start medication. Instead, the decision is based on your overall cardiovascular risk.

For people at highest risk (with existing cardiovascular disease), LDL cholesterol should usually be reduced to below 1.8 mmol/L (70 mg/dL), and sometimes even lower.

For people at high risk (primary prevention), statin therapy is recommended if your 10-year risk is 10 percent or higher (UK/Europe), with consideration for even lower thresholds in some cases.

For people at lower risk, lifestyle changes such as a heart-healthy diet, regular exercise, weight management, and smoking cessation are the mainstay of treatment. Medication may be considered if LDL remains very high despite these efforts, or if other risk factors are present.

Treating elevated fat levels with medication

If you and your doctor decide that medication is needed, statins remain the first-line treatment for most people. They effectively lower LDL cholesterol and have been shown to reduce the risk of heart attack and stroke. Ezetimibe or PCSK9 inhibitors may be added if targets are not met with statins alone.

Other medications, such as fibrates and nicotinic acid (niacin), are now rarely used for routine cholesterol management because they have not been shown to provide additional cardiovascular benefit beyond statins in most people. Bile acid sequestrants are also seldom prescribed today except in specific situations.

REMEMBER

Lifestyle changes — including a Mediterranean-style diet, regular physical activity, maintaining a healthy weight, and not smoking — are essential for everyone, regardless of your risk level or whether you take medication.

TIP

Recent research highlights that oxidized cholesterol and chronic inflammation are increasingly recognized as key drivers of cardiovascular risk, often providing a more complete picture than traditional cholesterol measures alone. While these factors are not yet routinely tested in clinical practice or included in standard risk calculators, both are strongly influenced by lifestyle choices such as diet and exercise, underscoring the importance of healthy habits for comprehensive heart protection.

Keeping Your Blood Pressure in Check

Keeping your blood pressure in check is essential, especially if you have prediabetes or diabetes. The rise in high blood pressure parallels the increase in these conditions, driven largely by increasing weight and sedentary lifestyles, a trend seen across all age groups.

But even if you've had your blood pressure taken hundreds of times before, do you actually know what the numbers mean? If you're concerned about high blood pressure but don't know what "high" actually means (or what numbers you should be aiming for), keep reading.

Clarifying the numbers

When someone checks your blood pressure, the result looks like this: 120/70 mmHg. What does this mean?

>> The upper (higher) number is called the *systolic blood pressure* and represents the force with which your heart expels blood into your arteries.

>> The lower (smaller) number is the *diastolic blood pressure* and represents the pressure in your arteries when your heart rests for a moment. Before that number can go lower, your heart begins to pump forcefully again.

>> Blood pressure measurements are described as mmHg (millimeters of mercury) because the earliest blood pressure measuring devices used the height of a column of mercury to indicate the pressure.

REMEMBER

Current guidelines define normal blood pressure as less than 120/80 mmHg. If your readings are consistently 130–139/80–89 mmHg, you have stage 1 hypertension, and levels of 140/90 mmHg or higher indicate stage 2 hypertension. For people with prediabetes or diabetes, the recommended target is now less than 130/80 mmHg — lower than in the past — because tighter control helps protect your heart, kidneys, and blood vessels from damage over time.

Dealing with high blood pressure

Lifestyle changes are the foundation of blood pressure management. Losing excess weight, increasing physical activity, reducing salt intake, and following a heart-healthy diet (such as the Mediterranean or DASH diet) can all make a significant difference. Stress-reduction techniques such as meditation and yoga may provide additional benefits, though their impact is generally smaller than that of diet and exercise.

If these measures fail, drug treatment can usually control your blood pressure. The numerous drugs available for treating high blood pressure fall into a few classes:

>> ACE inhibitors (for example, lisinopril, enalapril) and angiotensin receptor blockers (ARBs) (for example, candesartan, irbesartan) are often recommended first for people with diabetes or kidney disease, as they help protect the kidneys and reduce cardiovascular risk.

>> Calcium channel blockers (such as, amlodipine, nifedipine) and thiazide diuretics (for example, hydrochlorothiazide) are also commonly used, especially in older adults or Black individuals.

>> Beta blockers (such as, metoprolol) are now mainly reserved for specific situations, such as after a heart attack or in heart failure, rather than as routine treatment for high blood pressure.

>> Alpha blockers (such as doxazosin) are less commonly used as first-line treatment for high blood pressure today, except in specific situations, for example, in men who also have symptoms of an enlarged prostate. Diuretics (such as hydrochlorothiazide) are also prescribed less often as initial therapy than in the past but remain important for people with fluid retention or as part of combination treatment when blood pressure remains above target.

TIP

Medications may be chosen on the basis of preexisting conditions, contraindications and possibility of side effects. Combination therapy is often needed to reach your blood pressure target.

Looking for Evidence of Inflammation

Inflammation is now understood to play a central role in the development of prediabetes, Type 2 diabetes, and cardiovascular disease. C-reactive protein (CRP) is a blood test that reflects the level of inflammation in your body. Elevated CRP is common in people with prediabetes, metabolic syndrome, and diabetes, and is linked to a higher risk of developing these conditions as well as their complications.

CRP is more than just a marker, it may actively contribute to tissue damage, especially in the kidneys, where it can worsen inflammation and scarring through specific pathways. While CRP is strongly associated with cardiovascular risk, it is not routinely measured in everyone; it is most helpful for people at intermediate risk, where the result may influence treatment decisions.

According to the American Heart Association, CRP levels can be interpreted as follows:

>> **Low risk:** CRP less than 1.0 mg/L

>> **Average risk:** CRP 1.0–3.0 mg/L

>> **High risk:** CRP greater than 3.0 mg/L

Lowering CRP with lifestyle changes, such as weight loss, exercise, and quitting smoking can reduce your risk. Specific healthy dietary patterns such as the Mediterranean diet have been shown to reduce markers of inflammation including CRP. Statin medications, which lower both cholesterol and CRP, have been shown to reduce cardiovascular events, but CRP testing is not routinely used to decide who should take a statin.

Other tests for inflammation exist (such as the *erythrocyte sedimentation rate,* a measure of how fast your blood settles in a tube) but have not been proven very helpful. On the other hand, newer and more sensitive tests of inflammation, such as those that measure interleukin-6 (IL-6) or tumor necrosis factor (TNF), are becoming available. These tests are mostly used in research or specific medical conditions, but they reflect deeper levels of inflammation and may one day help assess risk more precisely than current tests such as CRP.

Hunting for Nutrient Deficiencies

In addition to water and sources of energy such as carbohydrate, fat, and protein, your body needs a variety of vitamins and minerals for good health. Fortunately, in the United States, most people get sufficient quantities of these substances in the food they eat. But there are exceptions, which we point out here.

Keeping your vitamin levels on target

You need a large number of vitamins in tiny quantities for good health. Table 6-1 lists the vitamins, their function, and the food sources that provide the largest amounts of them.

You can get most of these vitamins in the foods you eat, but specific diseases may correspond to a deficiency of each of the vitamins. See the book *Vitamins For Dummies* by Christopher Hobbs and Elson Haas (Wiley) for more information. If you and your doctor suspect that you may have a specific vitamin deficiency, you can have lab work done to check your blood levels of all these vitamins.

TIP

The one vitamin that should probably be measured much more frequently than all others is vitamin D. Scientists have found that vitamin D does a lot more than just help with absorption of calcium. Vitamin D is now considered similar to a hormone because it has effects all over the body. For example, vitamin D may protect against the following conditions:

>> Alzheimer's disease

>> Autoimmune arthritis

>> Cancer of the large intestine and breast

>> Cardiovascular disease

>> Diabetes

>> Multiple sclerosis

>> Stroke

Make sure you are getting enough vitamin D by having your doctor measure *25 hydroxy vitamin D.* Your level should be greater than 20–30 ng/mL. If not, you can take supplements in the form of vitamin D3 by mouth.

TABLE 6-1   **Vitamins You Need**

Vitamin	Function	Food Source
Vitamin A	Needed for healthy skin and bones	Milk and green vegetables
Vitamin B$_1$ (thiamin)	Converts carbohydrates into energy	Meat and whole grain cereals
Vitamin B$_2$ (riboflavin)	Needed to use food properly	Milk, cheese, fish, and green vegetables
Vitamin B$_6$ (pyridoxine), pantothenic acid, and biotin	All needed for growth	Liver, yeast, and many other foods
Vitamin B$_{12}$	Keeps the red blood cells and the nervous system healthy	Animal foods (for example, meat)
Folic acid	Keeps the red blood cells and the nervous system healthy	Green vegetables
Niacin	Helps release energy	Lean meat, fish, nuts, and legumes
Vitamin C	Helps maintain supportive tissues	Fruit and potatoes
Vitamin D	Helps with absorption of calcium, plus many other functions.	Dairy products, and it is made in the skin when exposed to sunlight
Vitamin E	Helps maintain cells	Vegetable oils and whole grain cereals
Vitamin K	Needed for proper clotting of the blood	Leafy vegetables, and it is made by bacteria in your intestine

Stocking up on minerals

Many minerals are also essential for good health. Table 6-2 lists the minerals, a summary of what they do, and how to obtain adequate amounts.

TABLE 6-2   **Minerals You Need**

Mineral	Function	Food Source
Calcium	For bones and teeth	Dairy
Phosphorus	For bones and teeth	Dairy
Magnesium	For bones and teeth	Dairy
Iron	Hemoglobin in red blood cells	Meat
Sodium	Regulates body water	Salt
Chromium	Stimulates fatty acids and cholesterol for brain function	Beef, liver, eggs
Iodine	For thyroid hormone	Salt, bread
Chloride, cobalt, zinc	Various functions	Lean meat, fish, nuts, and legumes

Your levels of these minerals can be measured, and you can take mineral supplements if necessary.

WARNING

It is possible to overdose on supplements and recommended to take the advice of a qualified and regulated health professional on which may be good (or potentially harmful) for you.

Certain groups are at higher risk of nutrient deficiencies, even in countries with generally good food supplies. Older adults, people with digestive disorders (such as celiac disease or Crohn's), those following strict plant-based diets, and individuals with limited sun exposure are particularly vulnerable, as are women of childbearing age (who are at risk for iron and folate deficiency) and young children (who may lack iron, vitamin D, or iodine). In addition, people with Type 2 diabetes often have a high prevalence of multiple micronutrient deficiencies, including some caused by side effects of medications used to treat diabetes. Socioeconomic factors also play a role, with lower income linked to poorer nutrient intake and higher risk of deficiency.

Getting a TSH test

The thyroid-stimulating hormone (TSH) test is a screening test for thyroid disease. Because thyroid disease often accompanies diabetes and thyroid disease tends to be asymptomatic, a TSH test is a good idea beginning at age 35. The test is also done on newborns to screen for low thyroid function. Prompt treatment with thyroid hormone can prevent loss of brain function. The test is done by measuring the TSH in a blood sample.

Chapter **7**

Children and the Elderly: Special Considerations

M uch of what we write in the rest of this book applies to all people, young and old alike. So why do we devote a special chapter to children and the elderly? The reasons are different for each:

» Children are growing and in a constant state of change. If that change involves putting on too much weight, the potential for future harm is great. Kids have a long time to develop complications if they progress to diabetes.

» The elderly have various medical conditions that complicate their health. Plus, they may have memory and learning problems that make caring for them more difficult.

If your child is putting on excess weight, take some of the steps we suggest in this chapter to reverse the situation as early as you can. Dealing with a few extra pounds early on is much easier than reversing a large weight gain that has been present for several years.

If you are elderly (over 70 years of age) or have an elderly parent, keep in mind that just growing older makes you more insulin resistant and more subject to prediabetes and diabetes. The suggestions in this chapter can help you delay or prevent the transition from prediabetes to diabetes and perhaps even return to the state of normal blood glucose metabolism.

Diagnosing and Managing Prediabetes in Children

Childhood obesity experts are discovering signs of diabetes, high blood pressure, high cholesterol, and liver disease in many children under the age of twelve.

In the United States, nearly 20 percent of children and adolescents aged 2 to nineteen are now classified as obese, and even more are overweight. These numbers have tripled since the 1970s and are increasing in many other parts of the world as well. According to the World Health Organization, more than 390 million children and adolescents aged 5 through nineteen were overweight in 2022, including 160 million living with obesity — a challenge that now affects countries at every income level. If this trend continues, many children today may face a shorter and less healthy future than their parents.

Before you concern yourself with reversing prediabetes or preventing Type 2 diabetes in your child, you need to know if they are overweight or obese. If you determine that they are, you want to know what to do. We cover these subjects in this section.

Checking if your child is overweight

In Chapter 6, we show you how to calculate your body mass index (BMI). For children, determining whether the BMI is a problem is more complex than for adults. That's because children are growing and may possibly grow out of the problem.

Children with a BMI from the 5th to the 84th percentile are considered normal in weight. Children are considered at risk for being overweight if their BMI is between the 85th and 94th percentile for height and weight. Obesity is defined as a BMI at or above the 95th percentile for height and weight. Because children are growing, a single BMI reading provides only part of the picture. What matters most is how their BMI changes over time, especially if weight gain outpaces growth in height.

TIP

An easy way to calculate your child's BMI percentile is to use online tools provided by trusted national health sources (the Centers for Disease Control and Prevention (CDC) in the United States, the National Health Service (NHS) in the UK, Diabetes Canada, or Australia's Department of Health). These calculators compare your child's BMI to others of the same age and sex, helping you understand whether they're in a healthy range for their population.

If your child is in the overweight category, they may grow out of it as they get older and taller. But they may not, which means that some change in their life-style is necessary. Your job is to check their BMI regularly over time to see if it gets better or worse. That information can help you determine what action to take.

If your child is in the obese range, taking action now is important. With your support, gradual and sustainable changes to eating habits, screen time, and physical activity can make a big difference to their long-term health.

Securing a diagnosis and taking action

For a child who is obese or who remains overweight, you need to find out whether prediabetes is present. When you get a diagnosis, the next step is to create an action plan. We cover both topics here.

Making the diagnosis in children

You must find out if your overweight or obese child has prediabetes already. The diagnosis is made the same way as it is for adults: by doing a *fasting blood glucose test* or a *glucose challenge*:

>> **Fasting blood glucose:** The lab checks your child's blood glucose levels after an overnight fast. A healthy child's test results are less than 100 mg/dL.

>> **Glucose challenge:** The lab checks your child's blood glucose two hours after they consume a calculated amount of glucose. The test results should be less than 140 mg/dL.

How much glucose does your child consume for this test? For each kilogram of body weight, they drink 1.75 grams of glucose. Say your child weighs 60 pounds. Your pediatrician divides that number by 2.2 to get the number of kilograms, which in this case is 27.3. Then they multiply that number by 1.75. They know to give your child 47.8 (or approximately 48) grams of glucose.

Many experts believe that the fasting blood glucose test misses too many children with prediabetes, and they prefer using the glucose challenge.

REMEMBER

For children, the oral glucose tolerance test (OGTT) is the most sensitive and reliable way to diagnose prediabetes, while the hemoglobin A1c (HbA1c) test though easier to perform and used routinely for adults, misses many cases and is not recommended as a stand-alone screening tool in this age group. While an HbA1c of 5.7–6.4 percent may suggest prediabetes in adults, this cutoff has poor sensitivity in children and should not be used alone to make the diagnosis.

Planning a lifestyle program

If your child has been diagnosed with prediabetes, what do you do next? We make several recommendations in Chapters 6 and 9, which we discuss at greater length in Part 5. But this list gets you started:

>> **Get your child's buy-in.** Work together as a family to set realistic, positive goals for eating and activity. Explain to your child in simple, age-appropriate ways how these changes help their body stay strong and healthy. When everyone is involved, healthy habits become easier to maintain and more likely to last.

>> **Begin a daily exercise program with your child.** Don't just direct your child to run and stand there with a stopwatch. What's good for them is good for you and good for your relationship. Make moving a fun, daily family activity — walk, bike, dance, or play sports together. Aim for at least 60 minutes of moderate-to-vigorous activity each day, and include muscle-strengthening exercises three times a week. When children see adults enjoying physical activity, they're more likely to join in and stick with it.

>> **Keep screen time under control.** Limit your child to two hours of looking at screens daily, which includes TV, computers, cell phones, video games, and so on. I'm not talking about time spent on the computer doing homework; that time can be excluded from the two-hour limit. I'm talking about nonessential screen time (although what you define as nonessential and what your child defines as nonessential may differ considerably).

>> **Stop going to fast food restaurants and to restaurants that offer buffets.** You may be able to return to those places after the problem is brought under control, but stay away for now.

>> **Eliminate ultra-processed foods and processed meats completely.** This includes salami and other luncheon meats, which are filled with chemicals that make people sick over time.

>> **Try to introduce a variety of vegetables and fruits as early as possible.** The earlier you do so, the more likely your child will eat and enjoy fruits and vegetables. Here are some specific ideas:

  ● Get fruits and vegetables into foods your child already likes, such as shakes, muffins, lasagna, soup, and omelets.

  ● Switch from soda to more healthy choices.

  ● Mix fruit with yogurt or your child's cereal.

- Make a snack of raisins, other pieces of dried fruit, and nuts.
- Serve vegetables as a stir-fry, made with minimal oil and use extra virgin olive oil.
- Start a vegetable garden with your child to enjoy the freshest possible produce.
- Go to a local farmers' market and let your child pick out the vegetables they want to eat.
- Start thinking of corn, potatoes, and rice as starches rather than vegetables. Your child should eat less of them.
- Eat plenty of vegetables yourself. Your child wants to imitate you.

REMEMBER

For a toddler, a serving of vegetables is much smaller than for an adult. The serving size is a tablespoon per year of age, so a 5 year old needs just 5 tablespoons per day (not five zucchinis). Past the age of 8, a serving size is a cup of raw vegetables, a half cup of cooked vegetables, or a whole fruit.

Treating your child if lifestyle change fails

If helping your child change their eating and exercise habits does not halt or reverse their prediabetes, you have other options:

>> **Medications:** As yet, the FDA and other regulatory organizations have not approved any medications specifically for prediabetes, but some medications can prevent prediabetes from becoming diabetes. Metformin in particular may be used "off license" by some doctors with specialist knowledge and in very high-risk patients.

>> **Bariatric surgery:** Surgery for obesity and to prevent diabetes in children is an extreme solution, but there are rare occasions when it may be performed as a last resort. The surgery is usually done when the child is an adolescent.

COMMUNITY-WIDE "THIN LIVING"

In 2004, communities throughout France launched an initiative called "Together, Let's Prevent Obesity in Children." The initiative was based on a successful program begun in two French towns between 1992 and 1997. The towns followed a healthy nutritional program to change children's eating habits. The initiative included special lessons in schools and colleges, the distribution of breakfasts, physician support, teacher

(continued)

(continued)

instruction on how to add healthy eating to the curriculum, and school visits by dietitians. Children in these two towns did not gain abnormal amounts of weight compared to other nearby towns, where they did. Families improved their eating habits.

The much larger program begun in 2004 initially included ten towns. Later, that number grew to 113 towns. The towns received suggestions for activities, diets, and community initiatives. Handouts were provided in shops and supermarkets. The towns created safe routes to walk to school, food professionals talked in the schools, and schools encouraged their students to exercise.

The results of the larger program have been encouraging. Obesity levels have fallen. Children are eating more nutritious food, and they are doing more exercise. The program is spreading to communities in Spain, Belgium, and other countries through the European Public Health Alliance.

This kind of community-wide program may be more successful in the long run than individual attempts to reduce obesity and improve food and exercise habits.

Paying Close Attention to the Elderly

George Bernard Shaw was once showing a friend a bust of himself that had been sculpted by the great painter Renoir. Shaw remarked, "It's a funny thing about that bust. As time goes on, it seems to get younger and younger." Unfortunately, at the present time, only our likenesses can stay young. But we can do plenty to slow down the processes of aging and developing illnesses (which could end the aging process as well).

REMEMBER

Today, about one in four adults over 65 in the US has diabetes, and more than half meet criteria for prediabetes, though the exact numbers depend on how prediabetes is defined. Because older adults often live with multiple chronic conditions, such as heart disease, high blood pressure, kidney disease, vision problems, joint issues, and frailty, their care requires special attention to complexity and individual needs.

Cognitive impairment, including memory and thinking problems is common in older age and can be worsened by prediabetes, diabetes, and obesity. This makes it essential to consider a person's ability to understand and follow a treatment plan. If someone cannot manage their care alone, involving family, caregivers, or community supports becomes vital for success.

Checking for memory and thinking disorders

As we grow older, changes in memory and thinking ability can become more common — and may be made worse by conditions like prediabetes, diabetes, or obesity. If cognitive issues are present, they can interfere with a person's ability to manage medications, follow a diet, or maintain a regular exercise routine. That's why screening for cognitive function is a key part of good care in older adults, particularly for anyone at risk of diabetes-related complications. Cognitive screening involves brief assessments designed to evaluate how well a person is functioning in areas such as memory, attention, problem-solving, language, and planning. These tools are not used to diagnose conditions like dementia on their own, but they help identify when further evaluation or support may be needed.

Two of the most commonly used and internationally validated tools are the Montreal Cognitive Assessment (MoCA) and the Mini-Mental State Examination (MMSE). Both take about 10 to fifteen minutes to complete and are widely used in clinics and hospitals around the world. They include tasks such as recalling lists of words, drawing a clock, performing simple calculations, naming objects, and answering orientation questions (such as the current date or location). These tests are easy to administer and provide helpful insight into whether someone may need additional medical attention or support in managing their day-to-day health.

If a person scores below the expected range, this may signal mild cognitive impairment or, in some cases, early signs of dementia. Follow-up assessments help track changes over time. When cognitive decline is detected, involving family members or caregivers in healthcare planning becomes especially important, so that the person gets the help they need to stay as independent and healthy as possible.

TIP

If you or a loved one are managing prediabetes or diabetes and are over 65, ask your doctor about cognitive screening during routine visits. Early detection of changes in memory or thinking can help tailor care and support to your needs.

REMEMBER

Cognitive screening tools such as the MoCA and MMSE are not diagnostic tests for dementia, but they are important first steps. If the results suggest a problem, further evaluation by a specialist — such as a geriatrician or neurologist — can help clarify the cause and guide next steps for care and support.

CONSIDERING KIDNEY FUNCTION

Age-related decline in kidney function may influence how the body handles glucose, though it is not a primary cause of high blood glucose. Blood flow to the kidney decreases by about 10 percent each decade after age 30 in a normal, healthy person. This decline may alter how the kidneys filter waste and metabolize certain drugs used to treat blood sugar and blood pressure. Circulation to the kidney is even less when high blood pressure or heart failure is present. Blood tests of kidney function may not reflect this decline because a key test measures the excretion of *creatinine,* a chemical that comes from muscle. With aging, muscle mass decreases along with the blood flow into the kidney, so less creatinine needs to be excreted and its level in the blood doesn't rise.

The main consequence of decreased blood flow to the kidney is the decreased ability of the kidney to get rid of salt, water, and glucose from the body. When the glucose rises to 180 mg/dL or higher, some is normally spilled into the urine. That process prevents the glucose from building up too high. The salt and water buildup causes the blood pressure to rise. Then the high blood pressure further decreases the kidney function. It's a vicious cycle.

Hormones coming from the adrenal gland, epinephrine and norepinephrine, are additional contributors to high glucose and blood pressure. Epinephrine raises blood pressure, heart rate, and blood glucose. Norepinephrine does the same thing. These hormones tend to be elevated in an elderly person's blood and don't fall as blood pressure rises.

Evaluating an elderly person's diet

If you don't live with the older adult you're supporting, you need to obtain a food history if at all possible because it represents such an important explanation for the development of prediabetes and diabetes. Ask the elderly person to write down *everything* they eat for three days. You may discover some of the following problems:

>> Little fresh vegetable and fruit intake

>> Little vitamin and mineral intake

>> An excess of highly processed carbohydrates such as cakes, candies, white rice, and white pasta

>> Too much red meat

>> Too much alcohol

You may want to steer them to a dietitian, who can develop a more balanced and lower calorie diet that's still enjoyable. Elderly people become less and less active with time, which is an important consideration in deciding how many calories someone should eat in a day.

Adding exercise to the program

Too often the elderly (especially the very elderly) do little or no exercise. This fact is very unfortunate because exercise not only prevents prediabetes in the elderly (just as it does in younger people) but also has a number of other benefits. For example, exercise:

>> Reduces the chance of a fall

>> Adds strength and stamina

>> Reduces the risk of high blood pressure

>> Decreases the resting heart rate, making the heart more efficient

>> Increases bone density to prevent fractures

>> Relieves constipation

>> Decreases stress

>> Improves mental function and delays dementia

The number of seniors is growing significantly — by 2030, one in five Americans will be older than 65. For this reason, a growing number of professionals specialize in working with the "active aging" population. Go online and type "Specialist for Active Aging" in your web browser to get an idea of what I'm talking about.

The elderly are often reluctant to exercise because they fear injury and pain in joints that already suffer from arthritis. They often don't realize that the opposite is true: By strengthening their muscles, they are able to function with less pain.

REMEMBER

Any older adult beginning a new or vigorous exercise routine should first consult their doctor. If a healthcare provider is hesitant about exercise, seek advice from another professional who supports safe physical activity for older adults.

Certain physical conditions may preclude doing aerobic exercise and resistance training:

>> A recent heart attack

>> Unstable chest pain

>> Heart failure

>> Uncontrolled high blood pressure

>> Uncontrolled metabolic disease, such as kidney or liver disease

Assuming these conditions don't apply and the doctor gives the green light to exercise, here are some guidelines for exercise in the elderly:

>> Exercise sessions don't have to be 30 minutes long. Three 10-minute sessions are just as good.

>> An elderly person (just like a younger person) should start slow and build up. They can walk just 10 minutes the first time, then twelve, then fifteen, and so forth.

>> Indoor training, especially on an exercise bike or an elliptical trainer, is just as good as outdoor exercise. Plus, these machines do not cause joint damage.

>> The elderly should do strength and resistance training, as well as aerobic exercise. In Chapter 17, I show examples of resistance training exercises, which require a small investment in a few light weights. Muscle strength declines by fifteen percent per decade after age fifty and thirty percent after age seventy, but resistance training can result in twenty-five to one-hundred percent strength gains in older adults.

>> Muscles grow stronger when they are overworked. The elderly should exercise to the point of muscle fatigue.

>> Excellent ways of improving balance are standing on one foot and then the other, walking heel to toe, or doing Tai Chi.

>> Someone who can't walk can still do exercises with their upper body, which can improve strength and stamina.

>> Meeting with an exercise trainer once or twice can ensure that the person is doing the exercises properly.

>> Walking in a pool is also an excellent way to exercise that minimizes the impact on joints while providing a satisfactory workout.

>> The elderly should exercise at the maximal intensity at which they can still carry on a conversation. That intensity increases over time.

Stopping the progression to diabetes

Preventing the progression from prediabetes to Type 2 diabetes in older adults involves thoughtful, personalized decisions. While the risk of diabetes increases with age, it's important to remember that prediabetes doesn't always progress and even modest lifestyle changes can significantly reduce that risk.

In later life, the goal isn't just adding years, but adding good years; maintaining independence, cognitive ability, and physical function. This means making adjustments that support healthy aging, not necessarily following the same strict interventions recommended for younger adults. For some older people, preventing frailty and falls may matter more than controlling glucose or HBa1C to a specific number.

The foundation of preventing diabetes is still lifestyle: regular movement, balanced meals with fewer ultra-processed carbohydrates, good sleep, and social engagement. Even small increases in physical activity like walking more often or doing simple strength exercises at home can improve insulin sensitivity and lower blood glucose. Eating patterns that emphasize vegetables, legumes, healthy fats, and whole grains (such as the Mediterranean-style diet) are linked to better metabolic and cardiovascular outcomes, even when followed in older age.

For those who are motivated and physically able, structured lifestyle programs, including weight loss or exercise plans may provide additional benefit. However, these should be adapted to the person's physical condition, energy levels, and priorities. What matters most is sustainability and how changes align with what the individual values in their daily life.

Medication is sometimes considered, especially when blood glucose levels are rising or when other risk factors such as cardiovascular disease are present. But the decision to start medication should weigh potential benefits (such as delaying or preventing diabetes) against possible side effects, cost, pill burden, and the person's overall health goals. Metformin is occasionally used in older adults at low doses, but it's not formally approved for prediabetes and isn't always necessary.

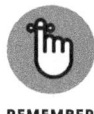

REMEMBER

Managing prediabetes in older adults is about shared decision-making helping each person understand their risk, reviewing the options, and choosing an approach that enhances both health and quality of life.

3

Food and Other Factors: Creating a Healthy Lifestyle

Chapter **8**

Setting Yourself Up for Success

With the abundance of processed and ultra-processed foods on the market and the extensive advertising campaigns used to promote them, many people have gotten away from buying, eating, and preparing real food. It is, however, the flavor and nutrients found in quality ingredients that can keep you both satisfied and on a healthful eating plan, and which will prevent prediabetes from turning in to Type 2 diabetes. If you're not used to eating and cooking with raw ingredients, it may seem daunting at first. But, equipped with the knowledge of how the food supply has changed and the benefits of healthy eating you can set yourself up for success in the kitchen and in life.

After you make a conscious commitment to eat healthfully, analyzing your kitchen and pantry is the first step to a rewarding future. Some of the food you have on hand may be very good for you, but if you live in an industrialized country, chances are that a lot of it should be put in the garbage, where it belongs, rather than in your body (or your child's body). How did we get to this state, where you are paying your hard-earned money for "foods" that hurt you? And I'm not talking about the constant food recalls that seem to be an everyday occurrence lately. Currently a lot of "ordinary" and "normal" food are available that you would do much better without.

In this chapter, we take a look at how our food supply got to the state it's in today. That food supply — along with our conversion from an active lifestyle to a sedentary lifestyle — is most responsible for promoting prediabetes and Type 2 diabetes.

While we're talking about food supply, we walk into your kitchen and pantry and point out the foods that belong there and the ones that don't. We explain why the rejected foods promote prediabetes.

Finally, we look at your child's lunchbox, as well as the food offered by the school for his lunch. Is that food contributing to your child's health or encouraging eating habits that will lead to disease and early death? Because healthy eating habits are so important in children, why not make them learn to love eating this way? We share the steps to take to help make this happen.

These are weighty matters, but isn't this discussion one of the reasons why you bought this book? You want to improve your health and set an example for your children. The information in this chapter can help you and your children develop healthy food habits that last a lifetime.

Understanding the Evolution of Our Food Supply

If we want to reverse our current epidemic of prediabetes and diabetes, we need to understand how we got here. And that requires knowing a little of the history of our food supply. After all, the kinds of foods that we consume tell us a lot about how we became so obese as a nation. So, get ready for an extremely condensed history lesson — one that will empower you to make the right choices.

Moving from forest to supermarket

We humans began as hunter-gatherers and continued to find our food in that way for thousands of years. We hunted for meat in the forest and found mushrooms there as well. We picked out the grasses that were tasty for our salads. We found wild fruits and berries on trees and bushes and ate those (not necessarily for dessert).

Believe it or not, some societies still live this way. They need to move from place to place as the food supply declines in one area and is available in another. This mobility has always tended to create a somewhat equal society because it's not possible to gather large amounts of possessions when you're constantly on the move.

The beginning of agriculture

About 10,000 years ago we started planting crops, and *agriculture*, or the science and practice of farming, began. Tribes could settle in an area and store some of the crops for the months when the weather did not permit growing food. In addition, it was becoming possible to keep animals to provide more food. With settlement, it became possible to accumulate possessions, which indicated someone's status in the society and which other members of the society coveted.

Some of the new farmers were particularly adept at growing large amounts of crops, and they became the sources of food for others who were more interested in creating things with their hands. Thus began the division of labor and the trading of food for other objects. With the invention of money, it became possible to hold the value of the food or object in a convenient way until it needed to be spent on something of similar value.

The introduction of artificial fertilizers

For centuries, farmers grew crops and maintained the fertility of their lands by mixing the manure of their animals into the soil. However, at the beginning of the 20th century a scientist discovered how to turn nitrogen, a key requirement for the growth of plants, from a gas into a solid that could be spread as a fertilizer. This process allowed farms to grow crops without having animals, and it erased the limitation on the size of the farm that results from the finite amount of animal fertilizer. For the first time, farmers could set up huge farms devoted to just one or two crops.

As cities began to fill up with people who were no longer needed on the farms because of advancements in farm machinery, large markets called *supermarkets* were established to provide their food. These markets preferred to do business with as few food providers (farmers and meat raisers) as possible, leading to even more concentration.

Corn for cattle

Some people believe that the root of our current obesity problem can be traced to 1973, when a new method of supporting corn farmers was established. The government incentivized farmers to plant as much corn as they possibly could. If the price of corn fell as a result, the US government would step in and pay the farmer directly. This situation led to an enormous supply of very cheap corn.

The people who raised cattle, chickens, and other animals, which had always been fed on grass, saw a way to raise more and fatter cattle, unlimited by the amount of grass available to them and using a source of very cheap calories. The animals could be concentrated in "feed lots," and their food would be brought to them instead of bringing them to the food (grass). The trouble was that cattle, especially, do not thrive when they eat a diet of corn or when they are concentrated together. They tend to get infections and have other problems that require antibiotics, so we end up eating those antibiotics. They also produce meat that is very fatty and filled with saturated fats, one of the worst kinds of fat.

Other abuses of corn

While some of the excess corn was being fed to cattle, plenty of corn was left. Food manufacturers saw this corn as an enormous source of cheap calories that they could use to produce new kinds of "food" products. They were able to put the sweetness of the corn into soft drinks, for example (most notably high fructose corn syrup, which we discuss in the next section). While they couldn't raise the price of normal-sized soft drinks (and actually, they should have lowered the price because corn sweetener is cheaper than sugar), they began to sell supersized bottles of soft drinks.

Food manufacturers were able to extract many compounds from the corn, which they put into other foods. Here are some of those compounds:

>> Corn oil

>> Citric acid

>> Lactic acid

>> Glucose

>> Fructose

>> Ethanol

>> Sorbitol

>> Mannitol

>> Xanthan gum

>> Modified and unmodified starches

>> Monosodium glutamate

You can find these ingredients on the labels of 10,000 to 12,000 of the 45,000 to 50,000 products found in the modern supermarket.

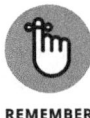

REMEMBER

Through advertising and promotion, food manufacturers strongly encourage you to eat foods containing these corn byproducts. These foods are cheap to make and significantly improve the manufacturers' bottom line. But these foods may also be pushing 200 to 300 extra kilocalories into your body every day. As a result, in one year you may gain 20 to 30 pounds.

Catering to our tastes

One of our favorite flavors is sweetness. Realizing this, food manufacturers have added sweetness in the form of high fructose corn syrup to just about everything. The problems are several:

>> We often don't know when to stop when we eat sweet foods because our natural ability to detect that we have eaten enough calories is bypassed by sweetness.

>> The foods that contain the increased sweetness are generally low in nutrition compared to foods such as fruits and vegetables. Food manufacturers really don't know what is missing from the foods they make, even when they add nutrients such as vitamins and minerals.

>> If we try to eat healthy by choosing items advertised as "low in fat," the sweetness in those foods can undermine our intentions. The excess carbohydrates turn to fat in our bodies.

>> The two largest sources of calories in the American diet, soft drinks and pastries, are made up largely of high fructose corn syrup.

Creating unrecognizable foods

Using all the components of corn, food manufacturers produce numerous products that are not actually foods but simply new combinations of those components. If you can't recognize something as food, it's not food. Just to give you an idea of what to look for so you can avoid it, here are a few examples of such products:

>> **Chili's Pepper Pals Country-Fried Chicken Crispers with Ranch Dressing and Homestyle Fries:** This item contains far too much salt, saturated fat, and calories.

>> **Keebler Fudge Shoppe Caramel Filled Cookies:** They're loaded with saturated fat, sugar, and calories.

>> **Kraft Cheez Whiz:** You get too much fat, salt, and calories.

>> **Tyson Chicken Breast Tenders:** They're filled with fat, saturated fat, salt, and calories.

>> **Kashi GOLEAN Oatmeal Raisin Cookie Bar:** Sounds almost healthy, right? But it's sweetened with enormous amounts of corn-derived sweeteners and has too much fat.

REMEMBER

Keep in mind that these are just a few of the processed foods that are not recommended as part of a healthy diet for anyone, let alone people with prediabetes. Labels are a great way to learn which types of ingredients are present in food. If you're going out to eat in a chain restaurant, you can often find out the ingredients and nutritional info by googling the menu choices prior to going to the restaurant.

Look at the ingredients (as provided by the manufacturer) of the last item on the list, the oatmeal raisin cookie bar, to give you the flavor of what constitutes food by the manufacturer's definition:

> Brown rice syrup *(a sweetener),* soy protein isolate *(the protein source),* evaporated cane juice crystals *(a sweetener),* crystalline fructose *(a sweetener),* Kashi seven whole grains and sesame blend, almonds, oat fiber, mechanically fractionated palm kernel oil, cocoa, rice flour, rice starch *(more carbs),* honey *(more carbs),* toasted soy grits, vegetable glycerin, corn grits, chicory root fiber, wheat bran, corn flour, natural flavors, salt, chocolate liquor, cocoa (with potassium carbonate), calcium carbonate, corn bran, magnesium oxide, soy lecithin, ascorbic acid, nonfat milk, vanilla extract, alpha tocopherol acetate, zinc oxide, ferrous fumerate, annatto, pyridoxine hydrochloride, folic acid, vitamin B12.

We recommend avoiding food with long ingredient lists as a whole but especially those with chemical sounding names. Is this food or a chemical concoction dreamed up in a laboratory? Wouldn't an apple or an orange do the trick just as well? We often hear people demonize fruit as having too much sugar or carbs, but the truth of the matter is that moderate quantities of whole foods are always better choices than processed snacks. See Chapter 15 for recipes and snack ideas. You know that Mother Nature has put all the ingredients for good health into those foods, and she requires no artificial coloring, flavoring, or excessive sweetness.

TIP

You could probably make a rule that anything with ten (possibly even five) or more chemical ingredients is not food. A second rule is to avoid foods that have ingredients with more than three syllables, such as *pyridoxine hydrochloride* — you don't need them added to your food.

Picking on Problem Ingredients

The previous section introduced you to the idea that problem ingredients abound in our food supply. Here, we want to talk specifically about some individual ingredients that you should avoid.

High fructose corn syrup

We bring up high fructose corn syrup several times in this book, with good reason. Because it's so cheap and satisfies our cravings for sweetness, food manufacturers use it in countless prepared foods. What are some of the principal problems with high fructose corn syrup?

» Any kind of sugar in excess is converted to fat in your liver — just what you don't want or need when you're battling prediabetes or diabetes.

» Fructose may actually make you feel *hungrier* as you eat more so you end up eating too many calories.

» Even if the sugar is not converted into fat, it's converted into glucose, which raises your blood glucose and further stresses your pancreas, possibly leading to prediabetes and diabetes.

» High fructose corn syrup is made from genetically modified corn, which is treated with genetically modified enzymes. If "genetic modification" is a dirty phrase in your vocabulary, avoid this ingredient.

» Fruit has fructose, but it also has fiber, which slows down its absorption. High fructose corn syrup lacks fiber.

» Your body can't tell the difference between types of sweeteners. If you give it something sweet, it will want more of it.

Given these and other problems associated with high fructose corn syrup, do you need to eat it? The answer is a resounding no!

Refined carbohydrates

Refined carbohydrates sound like something you should add to your diet. After all, who doesn't want to be more refined, or eat food that is more refined?

But the words are meant to confuse you. As carbohydrates are *refined*, all the good nutrients are removed. Refining means that the grain has been treated with machinery to strip away the bran and the germ from the whole grain. The bran and the germ contain the vitamins and the fiber so important to your health — the ingredients that lower your risk for diabetes, obesity, heart attacks, and high blood pressure.

Why do the food manufacturers refine carbohydrates? Oils in the grain germ become rancid after a while, so refined carbohydrates have a much longer shelf life than unrefined carbohydrates. But eating them definitely doesn't prolong *your* life! Refining is not beneficial for you — only for the food companies.

An interesting study in the *American Journal of Clinical Nutrition* in May 2004 showed that the increased consumption of refined carbohydrates such as high fructose corn syrup, along with the simultaneous decrease in fiber intake, paralleled the increase of Type 2 diabetes during the 20th century.

Here's how refined carbs really trip you up: You may think that a product such as sugar-free cookies is better for you than a product full of sugar. But the white flour in the cookies is rapidly broken down into glucose, which is rapidly absorbed in the absence of fiber and rapidly raises your blood glucose. So, we're sorry to disappoint you, but your sugar-free bakery products are not helping!

Following is just a partial list of refined carbohydrates and the common foods that contain them — items you should avoid:

>> White flour

>> White rice

>> Milled corn

>> Candy

>> Soda

>> Donuts and other pastries

>> Sweetened cereal

>> White bread

>> Granola

>> White pasta

The good news is that you don't have to be hungry. You just have to make good choices. Following are some of the foods you can substitute for those in the previous list:

>> Whole grains — barley, millet, quinoa, oats, whole wheat flour, and wheat berries

>> Beans, lentils, and peas

>> Nuts and other seeds

>> Vegetables

>> Fruits

>> Brown rice

The wrong types of fats

Fat is another word that has become almost profane. That's because we used to assume that the fat you ate would turn to fat in your body and clog your arteries. But not all fat is bad fat. Your body uses fat to make many important hormones such as estrogen, testosterone, and aldosterone. It's true that fat has more calories per gram than carbohydrate or protein, but it also enhances flavor. Fat can and should be a part of your diet if you keep the fat calories under control and emphasize the right fats. The different types of fat include:

>> **Saturated fat,** which is in animal sources of fat such as meat, butters, bacon, cream, and cream cheese. This fat increases levels of bad cholesterol and is much more prevalent in corn-fed cows than in grass-fed cows. Vegetable sources of more saturated (and therefore less healthy) fats are palm oil and coconut oil.

>> **Trans fats,** which are naturally present in very small amounts in foods but are a huge concern because of their *unnatural* presence in our food supply. Food manufacturers produce these fats by adding hydrogen to the next group of fats, the unsaturated fats. They use trans fats to replace butter, which is more expensive. But we now know that trans fats raise bad cholesterol and lower good cholesterol.

>> **Unsaturated fats,** which come from vegetable sources such as olive oil and canola oil. These fats are further broken down into two groups:

- *Monounsaturated fats* don't raise cholesterol in the blood. Olive oil is in this group. See Chapter 19 for more information on the benefits of good-quality extra virgin olive oil.

- *Polyunsaturated fats* don't raise total cholesterol but may lower good cholesterol. Examples are corn oil, mayonnaise, and some margarines.

Realizing that you want to emphasize monounsaturated sources of fat in your diet and minimize saturated fats, trans fats, and polyunsaturated fats is not hard. Fortunately, recent legislation is forcing the removal of trans fats from most foods.

Connecting Problem Foods to Prediabetes

How do problem foods encourage prediabetes and eventually diabetes? This section helps you understand why it's important to avoid them. The bottom line is that they promote obesity, which leads to prediabetes and diabetes, and they also increase the occurrence of heart disease.

Reacting to sugars and refined carbs

What happens in your body when sugars are absorbed? Why are refined carbohydrates and simple sugars so bad for you? This section gives you the complete picture of what's happening inside your body when you eat a cookie or a piece of cake.

Before table sugar (*sucrose*) enters your blood from your intestine, it's broken down into two sugars: glucose and fructose. When the glucose levels in your blood rise, the glucose passes through the *pancreas,* a small organ behind the stomach that has two major functions:

>> To provide digestive enzymes directly into the small intestine

>> To provide insulin directly into the bloodstream

Insulin is the hormone (chemical) that opens up cells so glucose can penetrate.

When you eat simple sugars such as sucrose and refined carbohydrates as in white flour, they are quickly broken down and quickly absorbed into your bloodstream. That's because there is little or no fiber or fat to slow down their absorption. They cause a rapid increase in the insulin levels in your blood. The result is that your cells take in glucose rapidly, and that glucose gets stored in your muscles and fat. Glucose is stored in the muscles in the form of *glycogen,* a long train of glucose molecules. In fat, glucose is stored as *triglyceride.*

REMEMBER

If your daily intake of calories is equal to or less than your daily expenditure, you burn up all this excess glycogen and triglyceride. If your daily intake is greater than your expenditure (which is the case for anyone who is obese), you store more of the excess glucose. The results are fatty changes in your liver (the presence of much more fat than normal in each liver cell), weight gain, and the development of blockages in your arteries that may lead to heart attacks, strokes, or *peripheral vascular disease* (the blockage of arteries to your legs).

As you gain weight, your body's insulin becomes less effective, and you have to release more of it from your pancreas to lower the blood glucose to the same extent. This condition is called *insulin resistance.* At some point, the pancreas can't keep up. You begin to have impaired fasting glucose and/or impaired glucose tolerance (conditions we describe in Chapter 1). At that point, you have prediabetes.

Unless the impairment is reversed by weight loss and exercise, the process worsens until you reach levels of blood glucose that define diabetes. When diabetes is present, you may develop the complications that we discuss in Chapter 3. (Sometimes, complications begin even before you reach a diagnosis of diabetes.) The tendency to develop heart disease begins even in prediabetes.

The continued overstimulation of the pancreas by high glucose levels can lead to the loss of pancreatic function and even higher glucose levels.

Realizing the consequences of eating bad fat

As we point out earlier in the chapter, there are good fats and there are bad fats. Good fats such as olive oil lead to improved blood flow through your arteries. Bad fats such as saturated fats and trans fats can cause your arteries to become blocked.

When arteries are blocked, you may develop coronary artery disease (*coronary* means "heart"), stroke, or peripheral vascular disease (due to the blockage of arteries to your legs).

In the last three decades, the number of deaths in the United States due to heart disease has fallen dramatically thanks to all kinds of new treatments, as well as improved diets. However, the tremendous increase in the number of Type 2 diabetes patients predicted for the next few decades may reverse this trend.

Stick to eating monounsaturated fats such as olive oil and canola oil if possible.

Another category of fats is called *fatty acids.* They're found in fish-like salmon, tuna, and halibut, as well as in nut oils and tofu. Another name for them is *polyunsaturated fatty acids.* The most important and healthful of this group are the omega-3 fatty acids. These fatty acids reduce inflammation and the risks of chronic diseases such as heart disease, cancer, and arthritis. Another group of fatty acids, the omega-6 fatty acids, promote inflammation.

The balance between omega-3 and omega-6 is important. You should consume two to four times as much omega-6 as omega-3. Most of us have no problem eating enough omega-6: Corn-fed cattle contain lots of omega-6, as do corn-fed farmed salmon. As a result, many people eat much more omega-6 than they need, and not nearly enough omega-3. This imbalance may explain the increase in inflammatory diseases in the United States. Taking omega-3 fatty acids in pill form may not provide the same protection.

Farm-raised salmon, fed on grain, may have an unhealthy ratio of omega-6 to omega-3 fatty acids. Stick to wild salmon.

Battling food cravings

Some physicians believe that harmful foods, especially sweeteners, stimulate chemicals in the brain (particularly a chemical called *dopamine*) that give an opiate-like feeling. You get "high" and want more of that feeling, so you eat more of that food.

Many doctors (including me) are skeptical that food could have the same potential for addiction as narcotics, alcohol, and sex. But how else do you explain the many people who eat large quantities of food that they know is hurting them? Doctors and others tell them to stop, but they continue to do it. Whether or not this eating behavior is based in addiction, it can be changed. Narcotics addicts, alcoholics, and sex addicts can control their behavior. And so can you if you feel that you fall into this category.

TIP

Try reducing or eliminating just one of the problem foods at a time. You'll find that you can actually live without it. If necessary, go for only a day without it and allow yourself to eat that food on the second day. Then try to skip two days, three days, and so forth. You'll be amazed at how long you can go without that food, and eventually you can give it up altogether.

When you first eliminate the offending foods, you may experience some symptoms such as headaches. Try to keep at it, and the symptoms will go away.

Becoming Aware of the Glycemic Index and Glycemic Load

The glycemic index is a controversial concept in nutrition. Many doctors believe it is important and helpful, but others and certain organizations (such as the American Diabetes Association) think it is too complicated for general use. I believe that the glycemic index provides important and helpful information. Even if that information is an approximation, you should understand how to use it.

The *glycemic index* (GI) is the degree to which a source of carbohydrate raises your blood glucose compared to white bread. White bread is assigned a value of 100. Another carbohydrate containing the same amount of calories is eaten, and blood glucose levels are determined and compared to the blood glucose levels found after eating white bread. Foods that raise the blood glucose half as much as white bread have a GI of 50, for example.

A study published in the *Archives of Internal Medicine* verified the usefulness of the GI. In one study from China, women who ate high GI rice had a significant increase in the risk of diabetes. Another study in the same journal showed a reduced risk of developing diabetes in black women who ate a diet that contained low glycemic cereal.

TIP

Select carbohydrates that have a low glycemic index if possible. You won't find refined carbohydrates in this category.

Some doctors are reluctant to use the GI more often for these reasons:

» Carbohydrates have different GIs if they're eaten alone or with other food.

» One food may have various GI counts depending on how it's processed or prepared.

» Certain low GI foods (for example, chocolate) contain a lot of fat.

» Diabetes educators are reluctant to teach about the GI because they believe it's hard to understand and creates confusion.

We believe the GI is a simple concept as long as we don't try to get too specific about numbers. We can simply suggest low glycemic substitutions for high glycemic foods and leave it at that. For example:

» Use whole grain bread rather than white bread.

» Eat unrefined whole grain cereal in place of processed breakfast cereal.

» Eat cookies made with dried fruits or whole grains instead of plain cookies.

» Eat cakes and muffins made with fruit, oats, and whole grains.

» Emphasize temperate climate fruits such as apples and peaches instead of warm climate fruits as in bananas.

» Eat whole wheat pasta or legumes such as beans and peas rather than potatoes.

» Use basmati or other low GI rice rather than white rice.

REMEMBER

Just because the GI is low (as in chocolate), that does not mean the food is good for you. Make sure you check the fat content before you make that food a major part of your diet. On the other hand, a food may have a high GI but may still be acceptable in a healthy diet if it contains very little carbohydrate. For example, a cantaloupe has a GI of about 70, but the amount of total carbohydrate is so low that it doesn't raise your blood glucose significantly when you eat a normal portion. This concept is called the glycemic load (GL), a number that takes both glycemic index and total carbohydrates into account. A GL of 20 is high, 11 to 19 is medium, and 10 or less is low. The glycemic load is perhaps more useful than the glycemic index because it measures the impact of combinations of foods when eaten together which more realistically reflects what happens when we eat a meal. Visit www.glycemicindex.com to discover more about GI, portion sizes, and GL.

Analyzing Your Child's Lunchbox and Lunchroom

Good eating habits must be developed at the earliest possible age. A child who is taught at home or at school that junk food and fast food are the normal diet will have a difficult time learning to eat a healthier diet later in life.

The lunches served in schools, other than a few exceptions, are becoming increasingly processed in the United States. While many schools use processed foods that go from freezer to lunch tray, others have cafeterias that heat up the processed food before serving it to children. These items traditionally include unhealthy versions of processed spaghetti, macaroni and cheese, hamburgers, peanut butter and jelly sandwiches, and chicken tenders. Parents often report problems with the quality and freshness of these foods.

Just making the previously mentioned items from scratch is a step in the right direction. If you can take the extra time to make the children's lunches, or have someone do it for you, they are better off. This way you can take control of what your children eat to save them from having further health risks in the future.

Checking the lunchbox

What do you put in your child's lunchbox? A sandwich made of white bread, mayonnaise, and luncheon meats? Or a salad with tofu and various fruits and vegetables? After reading this chapter, you should have a pretty good idea of what to send in that lunchbox. Here are some specific suggestions:

» Bento boxes filled with hummus, crudites, whole wheat pita and crackers, or whole wheat crackers, olives, nuts, cheese, and fresh fruit, or hard boiled eggs, guacamole, baby carrots, celery, whole wheat pita or crackers

» A green salad with protein such as chicken, eggs, tofu, or fish

» Whole grain bread sandwiches with real chicken, tuna, or eggs

» Quesadillas or wraps made with homemade tortillas, fresh vegetables such as corn, mixed peppers, lettuce, black beans, chicken, and so forth

» Bean and vegetable bowls with brown rice or quinoa

» Falafel pita pockets

» Whole wheat pasta salad dressed with extra-virgin olive oil and veggies

» Fresh fruit salad including grapes, blueberries, apples, or other seasonal fruit

- >> Nuts including almonds, cashews, or walnuts

- >> Baby carrots

- >> Raw green beans, broccoli, snap peas, or cauliflower with an EVOO/lemon juice vinaigrette for dipping

- >> Vanilla-flavored Greek yogurt

- >> A container of plain milk

In other words, give them whole grains, beans, nuts and other seeds, vegetables, and fruits. Avoid processed foods with more than five ingredients that have more than three syllables in their name!

If your child has been eating healthy foods at home, you shouldn't have a hard time getting him to eat the same way at school. They already know that they enjoy these foods, and they may even be eager to teach their friends what they know about nutrition.

Looking at school lunches

Unfortunately, most middle schools and high schools have vending machines that are filled with junk such as soda, imitation fruit juices, candy, chips, and cookies. And if your child eats a lunch prepared in the school cafeteria, they may not do much better. School lunches often feature pizza, hot dogs, french fries, chips, cookies, and other processed and prepared foods.

The US government pays for what's called the National School Lunch Program (NSLP), but the money isn't used to increase our kids' nutrition. Instead, most of the money goes for non-food items such as heating the cafeteria. Foods distributed by the NSLP contain many of the same ingredients as the vending machines; they do not make up a nutritious meal.

For some school nutrition success stories, go to the Web site `https://www.cdc.gov/school-nutrition/about/?CDC_AAref_Val=https://www.cdc.gov/healthyschools/nutrition/schoolnutrition.htm`. You may be inspired by what other parents have achieved in the lunchroom.

The bottom line: Don't leave your child's hot lunch choices up to the school. Find out for yourself what your child is eating in school and improve everyone's diet by using what you have discovered in this chapter to encourage good nutrition.

Making healthy foods enticing for kids

Some "ingredients for life" children crave more than unhealthy foods. It is actually the love and attention of their parents that nourishes them the most. As you begin to embark on a healthier eating journey with your children, think about additional ways to spend time with them, and show them your affection.

Here are some ways to spend more time with kids while helping them to eat better:

1. **Get your kids involved in meal planning** — talk about dishes that they like which you know are good for them — or ideas that you have in mind.

2. **Try planting a garden,** if you have the room. Send some of the produce with your child. They will be proud to show their friends that they and you grew this food. Plus this food is the freshest and most nutritious food they can eat.

3. **Plant a flower box** or some pots on a windowsill with fresh herbs, garlic, and chili peppers. Ingredients such as these grow anywhere, give children the pleasure of taking care of plants, and produce antioxidant rich ingredients.

4. **Be sure that kids know that you're making these changes because you love them and prioritize their health.**

5. **Bring kids to farms and the farmers market,** or the produce section of a grocery store and ask them what they'd like to try.

6. **Create new recipe ideas together!**

7. **Get the kids in the kitchen** to help with cooking and serving — give them lots of compliments and positive feedback.

8. **Start new traditions such as theme nights** — (Healthy) Taco Tuesday, Pizza Saturday, and so forth that enables them to eat and make better versions of foods that they love.

9. **Bake wholesome and diabetes-friendly desserts** with them. See *Diabetes Desserts For Dummies* by Amy Riolo for ideas.

With the right intentions and a few strategies up your sleeves, you can help change your child's eating habits for the better. Staying clear of food problems, avoiding cravings, and fueling your appetite for creating healthy meals for yourself and your family can help you to stop the progression from a prediabetes to a diabetes Type 2 diagnosis easily and effectively. Plus, a better diet improves other areas of your health, your appearance, and your overall well-being.

Chapter **9**

Achieving and Maintaining a Healthy Weight

Among the most important reasons to monitor prediabetes is that it often progresses to Type 2 diabetes, a condition that can lead to serious complications, including heart disease, stroke, kidney disease, eye problems, and even dementia. Worryingly, even when blood sugar levels are only slightly higher than normal, as they are in prediabetes, the risk of developing some of these chronic conditions already begins to rise.

Prediabetes develops mainly because of insulin resistance, which means the body's cells become less responsive to insulin. This reduced efficiency causes blood glucose levels to climb above the healthy range. Many factors can contribute to insulin resistance, including genetics, age, certain medications, and medical conditions that affect hormone levels and interact with insulin, such as Cushing's disease or polycystic ovary syndrome (PCOS). Chronic stress and poor sleep can also play a role.

However, the most significant contributors are excess body weight, an unhealthy diet, and a lack of physical activity. The good news is that these interrelated factors are issues that we can do something about.

This chapter explores body weight and its relationship with prediabetes.

Benefitting from a Healthy Weight

Carrying excess weight is one of the important factors contributing to insulin resistance, especially when that weight is centered around the abdomen. Abdominal fat, more than fat stored elsewhere, releases inflammatory chemicals and hormones that interfere with insulin's function. This makes it harder for your body to move sugar out of your bloodstream, leading to higher blood glucose levels and raising the risk for prediabetes and eventually Type 2 diabetes.

A landmark clinical trial called the Diabetes Prevention Program (DPP) demonstrated just how effective weight changes can be. In this large, well-conducted study, adults with prediabetes who lost just five to seven percent of their body weight through better eating and regular physical activity reduced their risk of developing Type 2 diabetes by an impressive 58 percent over about three years, compared to a control group.

Considering how weight, diet, and exercise relate

Exercise, healthy eating and your body weight each play their own powerful, independent roles in reducing insulin resistance.

Physical activity helps your muscles use up glucose, improving how your body responds to insulin even if you don't lose weight. Diet also matters because eating a diet rich in fiber, healthy fats, and plant-based foods (such as the Mediterranean diet) can reduce inflammation, enhance insulin sensitivity, optimize glucose levels and lower the risk of developing prediabetes and diabetes.

Importantly, lifestyle changes with the Mediterranean diet provide benefits far beyond weight loss alone. The PREDIMED study, a major Spanish clinical trial, found that people who followed a Mediterranean diet were 52 percent less likely to develop Type 2 diabetes, even if they didn't lose any weight. In other words, making changes to what you eat can dramatically lower diabetes risk regardless of the number on the weighing scale.

A study from Uppsala University published in 2020 followed over 79,000 individuals for over 20 years. It found that high adherence to a Mediterranean diet substantially mitigates the increased risk of all-cause mortality typically associated with being overweight or obese, so much so that overweight or obese people following this diet had mortality rates similar to or even lower than their normal-weight counterparts with low diet adherence. Overall, the study demonstrates that diet quality, particularly adherence to a Mediterranean-like pattern, can largely compensate for the risks of raised BMI in terms of longevity, highlighting its importance above BMI alone for long-term health outcomes. Even though this particular study did not specifically look at prediabetes and diabetes, it's an important lesson in the placing a high value on diet quality, especially for those people who struggle to lose weight.

The bottom line is that positive changes in diet and physical activity can help you lose weight but each also helps your body use insulin more efficiently and can dramatically lower your risk of progressing to prediabetes and from prediabetes to Type 2 diabetes. The benefits of a healthy lifestyle go well beyond weight, making you healthier from the inside out.

REMEMBER

You will probably be at the lowest risk of developing prediabetes if you have a normal weight. Exercising regularly and having a Mediterranean-style diet may well help you achieve your optimum weight but if that doesn't happen it is important to appreciate that you become much healthier, with reduced risks of prediabetes, diabetes, and other serious illnesses by adopting these lifestyle changes irrespective of your body weight. On the other hand, if you have a poor-quality diet, you will be at increased risk of diabetes as well as many other chronic diseases even if you are of normal weight.

Defining a healthy weight

Being more active and improving your diet can make you metabolically healthier on many levels, by lowering blood sugar, reducing inflammation, and improving cholesterol and blood pressure, even if the scale doesn't move much. These factors are also closely connected.

Exercise and a Mediterranean-style diet can support weight loss, but when you combine exercise, an excellent diet and an optimum weight, you benefit from the greatest benefits of all.

We explore how to get more exercise and enjoy a Mediterranean-style diet, both of which have been shown to support achieving and maintaining a healthy weight as well as separately improving glucose regulation by reducing insulin resistance in later chapters. In the sections that follow, we consider how to assess your weight and how you can aim for a healthy body size.

Becoming Familiar with Your Body Mass Index

Here's an interesting question: How can four people who all weigh 125 pounds be classified as underweight, normal weight, overweight, and obese? The answer lies in their *height*. Weight alone doesn't tell us enough — it's how your weight relates to your height that determines where you fall on the Body Mass Index (BMI) scale.

For example:

>> A man who is 5'8" and weighs 125 pounds would be considered underweight.

>> A woman who is 5'3" and weighs the same would fall within the normal weight range.

>> A person who is 4'10" and weighs 125 pounds would be classified as overweight.

>> And someone who is 4'6" tall at that weight would fall into the obese category.

These examples highlight why BMI is used as a basic screening tool. It combines height and weight to give a general sense of whether someone may be at increased risk for health problems related to body fat. You can calculate your BMI by using this formula:

1. Multiply your weight in pounds by 703.

2. Divide that number by your height in inches.

3. Divide again by your height in inches.

For instance, if you are 5'4" (64 inches) and weigh 125 pounds:

$125 \times 703 = 87,875$

$87,875 \div 64 = 1,373$

$1,373 \div 64 = \mathbf{21.5}$

A BMI of 21.5 falls within the "normal" range.

The BMI categories are:

>> **Underweight:** less than 18.5

>> **Normal weight:** 18.5 to 24.9

>> **Overweight:** 25 to 29.9

>> **Obese:** 30 and above

You can also calculate your BMI quickly using reliable online tools, such as the CDC's calculator:

`https://www.cdc.gov/bmi`. **Table 9-1 shows a Body Mass Index chart distribution shows BMI scores based on weight and height.**

While BMI can be a useful starting point, understanding its limits is important. It doesn't measure body fat, account for muscle mass, or reflect differences between individuals due to age, sex, ethnicity, or body composition. A very fit person such as a rugby or football player may have a high BMI due to muscle, while someone with a "normal" BMI may still carry unhealthy levels of visceral fat. This is explored in more detail in the next section.

That's why BMI should never be used as a judgment of health in isolation. It's one tool among many, including waist circumference, blood tests, physical activity, diet and lifestyle and overall well-being, to help build a fuller picture of someone's health.

In the past, some guidelines included simplified formulas to estimate "ideal weight" by height and gender. For example, 106 pounds for five feet tall in men, plus six pounds for each inch over that, or 100 pounds for women plus five pounds per inch. But these formulas don't reflect the wide range of healthy body types and are rarely used in modern health assessments.

REMEMBER

Ultimately, the goal is not to hit a specific number on the scale, but to support overall health, through balanced nutrition, physical activity, sleep, stress management, and self-care, in a way that's sustainable and respectful of your body.

TIP

In older adults, having a BMI in the "overweight" range (25–29.9) is often not only safe but may actually be associated with a lower risk of death compared to those in the "normal" weight range. This was highlighted in a major review published in the *Journal of the American Medical Association* (*JAMA*) in 2013, which pooled data from nearly 100 studies and over 2.8 million adults. The researchers found that, while obesity (BMI of 30 or more) was linked to higher mortality, individuals in the overweight range had a slightly lower risk of death than those in the normal range, and this effect was particularly noticeable in people aged 65 and older. One possible explanation is that older adults naturally lose muscle and bone mass over time, and a slightly higher body weight represent more muscle and bone density as well as providing protective nutritional and energy reserves during illness, surgery, or recovery from injury. In practical terms, this means that older individuals do not necessarily need to aim for a BMI in the "normal" range. Instead, maintaining strength, mobility, and good nutrition is more important than focusing solely on weight loss or BMI targets in later life.

TABLE 9-1 **Body Mass Index Chart**

Body Mass Index (kg/m²)	19	20	21	22	23	24	25	26	27	28	29	30	35	40
Height (Inches)	Weight (Pounds)													
58	91	96	100	105	110	115	119	124	129	134	138	143	167	191
59	94	99	104	109	114	119	124	128	133	138	143	148	173	198
60	97	102	107	112	118	123	128	133	138	143	148	153	179	204
61	100	106	111	116	122	127	132	137	143	148	153	158	185	211
62	104	109	115	120	126	131	136	142	147	153	158	164	191	218
63	107	113	118	124	130	135	141	146	152	158	163	169	197	225
64	110	116	122	128	134	140	145	151	157	163	169	174	204	232
65	114	120	126	132	138	144	150	156	162	168	174	180	210	240
66	118	124	130	136	142	148	155	161	167	173	179	186	216	247
67	121	127	134	140	146	153	159	166	172	178	185	191	223	255
68	125	131	138	144	151	158	164	171	177	184	190	197	230	262
69	128	135	142	149	155	162	169	176	182	189	196	203	236	270
70	132	139	146	153	160	167	174	181	188	195	202	207	243	278
71	136	143	150	157	165	172	179	186	193	200	208	215	250	286
72	140	147	154	162	169	177	184	191	199	206	213	221	258	294
73	144	151	159	166	174	182	189	197	204	212	219	227	265	302
74	148	155	163	171	179	186	194	202	210	218	225	233	272	311
75	152	160	168	176	184	192	200	208	216	224	232	240	279	319
76	156	164	172	180	189	197	205	213	221	230	238	246	287	328

Identifying Where You Carry Your Fat

Not all body fat is the same, and where you carry it makes a big difference to your health. Experts now distinguish between subcutaneous fat, the type just under the skin that you can pinch on your belly, hips, arms, or thighs, and visceral fat, which lies deeper in the abdomen and wraps around internal organs such as the liver and pancreas. While subcutaneous fat is more visible, visceral fat is far more dangerous, as it increases the risk of serious conditions such as Type 2 diabetes, heart disease, high blood pressure, metabolic syndrome, and even some cancers.

Putting on (or off) visceral fat

A well-known study from the Mayo Clinic, presented at the American Heart Association's Scientific Sessions in 2007, remains widely cited and relevant today. It found that even a modest weight gain of just 9 pounds in lean, healthy young adults caused a significant increase in visceral fat and impaired the function of blood vessels. In contrast, blood flow remained normal in those who maintained their weight. Importantly, when the participants who had gained weight lost it again, their blood vessel function returned to normal. This showed that even small increases in visceral fat can have early health effects, but also that these effects are reversible with modest weight loss.

As people age, it's natural for body fat to increase, and for more of it to settle around the abdomen — especially in women after menopause, due to hormonal changes. A lack of physical activity, poor quality diet, and excess energy intake all encourage visceral fat accumulation, but the good news is that this type of fat is also the most responsive to lifestyle changes. Regular physical activity, particularly aerobic exercise such as brisk walking, and a good diet can help reduce visceral fat even without major changes in overall weight.

Estimating your visceral fat

A practical way to assess whether you may be carrying too much visceral fat is to measure your waist circumference. In general, a waist size greater than 35 inches (88 cm) for women or 40 inches (102 cm) for men is associated with increased health risks. People of Asian heritage are at risk at lower thresholds — typically 31.5 inches (80 cm) for women and 35 inches (90 cm) for men — because they are more likely to store visceral fat even at lower body weights.

Another useful measure is your waist-to-height ratio, which compares the size of your waist to your height. To calculate it, divide your waist measurement by your height (both in the same units — inches or centimeters). A healthy ratio is less than 0.5, meaning your waist should be less than half your height. This method is gaining popularity because it adjusts for different body builds and is a good predictor of visceral fat and related health risks across different ages and ethnic groups.

The best news is that visceral fat is often the first to decrease when you adopt healthier habits. Losing just 5 to 10 percent of your body weight can significantly reduce visceral fat and improve key health indicators. Focusing on reducing waist size, rather than chasing a particular weight, can be a more meaningful and motivating way to protect your health, especially as you age.

Realizing How You Got Here

If you're overweight, you probably have spent many years getting to your current condition. In this section, I explore some of the routes you may have taken during those years. Understanding each one can provide you with the opportunity to change to a healthier lifestyle. Adding up all the changes can get you back to a body that promotes good health rather than the health risks we discuss in the previous section. Remember: When you feel great, that's when you can hit a home run!

Losing weight, and keeping it off, is not easy. Many people struggle despite genuine effort, and the reasons are both biological and environmental. Our bodies are wired to resist weight loss. When weight is lost, metabolism often slows down and hunger hormones increase, making it harder to maintain lower weight. This is not a failure of willpower — it's a protective survival mechanism. On top of this, the modern food environment, high in calorie-dense processed foods and shaped by convenience and marketing, makes it very difficult to make consistent healthy choices.

It's also important to recognize that attempts to shame people into losing weight are not only unkind but counterproductive. Studies show that weight stigma and negative self-image can actually increase the risk of unhealthy eating patterns, discourage physical activity, and worsen metabolic health. Encouraging sustainable, health-focused changes, rather than simply aiming for a number on the scale, is more effective and respectful.

Successful, long-term weight management is most often achieved through gradual, manageable lifestyle changes. This means focusing on a nourishing, balanced diet, incorporating more physical activity in enjoyable ways, and setting realistic goals. It also involves addressing stress, sleep, and emotional well-being, all of which play a role in weight and blood sugar regulation. With compassion and support — rather than criticism — people are far more likely to find a path to better health that they can maintain.

Considering calories

A *calorie* is a unit of energy. When we talk about calories in food, we're referring to the energy our bodies can extract and use from what we eat. Most adults need somewhere between 1,800 and 2,500 calories per day, depending on age, sex, body size, and activity level. If we regularly consume more calories than we use, the excess energy is stored in the body as fat, which over time can lead to weight gain.

This basic principle of energy in versus energy out underpins many approaches to weight management. However, it is not quite as simple as this. Your body does not simply add up the calories you have used through your daytime activities, subtract this from the calories you have eaten that day, and put the excess around your waist.

While calorie balance matters, and we refer to calories in this book, especially when we talk about the numbers of calories in large portion restaurant meals, not all calories are equal in how they affect hunger, hormones, metabolism, and long-term health. For example, fat contains more than twice the calories per ounce or gram compared to carbohydrates or protein, but this doesn't mean that low-fat diets are necessarily more effective for weight loss. In fact, fat can help increase satiety, improve blood sugar control, and support the absorption of important vitamins. Similarly, 100 calories from sugar-sweetened soda affect the body very differently than 100 calories from nuts or legumes. The type of food, its nutrient composition, how it's processed, its effect on the gut microbiome and even the order in which it's eaten can all influence how full you feel, how much insulin you release, and how much energy you ultimately store or burn. In short, calories count, but context counts more. Understanding the quality of what you eat is just as important as the quantity.

TIP

If you eat a balanced, healthy, unprocessed diet such as a Mediterranean diet, it is entirely possible, with modest portion sizes and mindful eating, to ignore the calorie content and to successfully lose weight.

Eating out

Eating out can be a real challenge, especially in fast food restaurants, those that offer "all you can eat" buffets, or where the eatery prides itself on the quantity of food in its servings.

Noting the problems you run into

Numerous issues make eating out difficult. Here are a few:

>> You have no idea what's in the food, and studies show that we generally underestimate the calories in restaurant food.

>> The meal may be delayed, and you may end up eating and drinking in the bar before the meal.

- » Restaurant portions, especially in the United States, are almost always too large.

- » Many easy-to-order foods take hours to prepare so people order them in restaurants instead of making them at home.

- » The descriptions of the foods on the menu, especially the desserts, make them hard to resist.

- » Hamburgers, french fries, and pizza are the top three US favorites for eating out.

Preparing to go to a restaurant

You can do several tasks before you get to the restaurant to decrease your chances of overeating:

- » Look at the menu online and make choices before you get to the restaurant. You are much more likely to make good choices this way.

- » Feel free to choose any type of ethnic food but avoid buffets.

- » Consider a local restaurant so you can walk to it and burn some calories on the way.

- » Find out if the restaurant has special meals for people who want to control their calories.

- » Drink water or have a vegetable snack before you go, to lessen your appetite.

- » Call and find out if the restaurant allows you to substitute lower calorie choices (such as a vegetable) for higher calorie choices (such as french fries). For example, the restaurant may:

  - Provide skim milk instead of whole milk

  - Reduce the amount of butter, sugar, and salt in a dish

  - Serve dressings and gravies on the side

  - Bake, broil, and poach rather than fry or sauté

Keeping your control at the restaurant

After you arrive at the restaurant, take these steps to reduce your risk of eating too much:

- » Don't arrive early. If you do, you may sit in the bar and order a drink (and snack on the salty items you find there).

>> Tell the host you need to be seated promptly.

>> Keep bread off the table if possible.

>> Ask for raw vegetables as you wait for the food.

>> Plan to take half your food home.

>> Order wine by the glass and have only one.

>> Remind yourself that soup and salad can make a delicious low-calorie meal.

>> Keep in mind that a vegetarian dish may not necessarily be good for you. It may contain a lot of processed ingredients just like the non-vegetarian option. Check it out by asking the waiter.

Miscalculating portions

Restaurant rule #1: The portions of food on your plate are always more than you should eat, often by a factor of two. If you eat half of what they serve you, you are probably eating the right amount. You can eat the other half at home the next night, and the meal actually costs half as much!

Why are restaurant portions so large? Restaurants supply what diners demand. Americans want a lot of food on their plates — much more food than European diners want, for example.

And because we're so used to seeing heaping portions of food when we dine out, our ideas about portion sizes get skewed even when we're preparing our own food at home. After all, if the restaurant offers a half-pound burger, why would you make anything smaller when you're grilling in your backyard?

But, of course, we *should* make something smaller at home. No one needs to consume 8 ounces of beef at one sitting, or four slices of bread, or a heaping pile of potatoes . . . We simply don't need so much food on our plates.

So what *do* you need on your plate at mealtime? Let me start by making some comparisons between ideal food portions and other objects that you can easily visualize:

TIP

>> Three ounces of meat, fish, or poultry is the size of a pack of cards.

>> A medium fruit is the size of a tennis ball.

>> A medium potato is the size of a computer mouse.

>> An ounce of cheese is the size of a domino.

>> A cup of fruit is the size of a baseball.

>> A cup of broccoli is the size of a light bulb.

Misreading your appetite and fullness

One common reason that people eat too many calories is they misread their appetite. Your appetite is a very subjective feeling. The definition of appetite is the desire to eat food, felt as hunger. The purpose of your appetite is to regulate your energy intake. If you already have large amounts of stored energy, you shouldn't have an appetite. Yet most often, you still do.

When you begin eating, your stomach gradually fills and stretches, and this triggers signals to the brain via hormones such as cholecystokinin (CCK), glucagon-like peptide-1 (GLP-1), and others. These hormones help slow stomach emptying and promote a sense of satisfaction (satiety). But this process takes time, typically 15 to 20 minutes or more. If someone eats quickly, they may consume more food than they need before these satiety signals have had a chance to kick in.

TIP

Eating slowly and mindfully is often recommended as a practical strategy to support healthy eating habits. By slowing down, chewing thoroughly, and pausing during a meal, you give your body time to process the food and communicate its signals of fullness more effectively. This approach can help reduce overeating and may support better weight management and blood sugar control, particularly in people with prediabetes or insulin resistance.

REMEMBER

Most hunger is habit, especially if you are overweight. If you simply ignore the sensation of hunger, you'll likely not experience any bad consequences.

Craving the wrong kinds of foods

If we would just crave carrots and celery, none of us would have any weight problems. Unfortunately, we usually crave stuff like doughnuts and chocolate. And if you give in to the craving and indulge in the doughnut or chocolate, your blood glucose rises. Then your body's insulin rises in response, sometimes sending your blood glucose too low, creating hunger. To appease the hunger, you eat more doughnuts or chocolate, of course.

We can break food cravings into two types:

>> **Psychological cravings:** These cravings reflect what you want, not what you need. They spur emotional eating.

>> **Physiological cravings:** These cravings reflect what you need. Your body is actually low on energy and has no stored supplies of carbohydrates or fats.

Most craving is psychological. When you eat sweets, your body releases a chemical called *serotonin* in your brain, which makes you feel happy. That's why certain sweets such as chocolate have come to be associated with positive emotions like love.

You can overcome these cravings for the wrong kinds of food. Here are a few tips:

TIP

>> Eat more protein.

>> Eat high fiber foods, including whole grains.

>> Don't eat refined foods such as white rice, white flour, or refined sugar.

>> Eat small, frequent meals (such as every three hours).

>> Wait for the craving to go away without feeding it.

>> Get plenty of exercise.

>> Don't skip meals.

>> Get enough sleep.

>> Occasionally allow yourself a little of what you crave.

Knowing That You Can Lose Weight

The best diet for managing prediabetes should help address one of its most significant risk factors — excess body weight — by supporting healthy, sustainable weight loss and optimum weight maintenance. Beyond weight, it should also help reduce insulin resistance, improve blood glucose regulation, and lower the risk of other chronic diseases. Importantly, it must be enjoyable, nutritionally balanced, and practical enough to maintain in the long term. The Mediterranean diet, which is explored in more detail in later chapters, meets all of these criteria. Rather than being a short-term or restrictive plan, it represents a long-term, sustainable way of eating that forms part of a broader healthy and active lifestyle.

Choosing the Mediterranean diet

The Mediterranean diet has consistently been shown to help people reach and maintain a healthy weight. Unlike many fad or restrictive diets, it is both effective and sustainable. Clinical studies have found that when this way of eating is combined with modest calorie and portion size control, people tend to lose weight, especially those who start with a higher body mass index (BMI). These weight reductions are often accompanied by improvements in blood pressure, cholesterol levels, insulin sensitivity, and inflammation — all important markers of metabolic health.

In a recent 12-month study comparing different popular approaches, including intermittent fasting and daily calorie counting, people following a Mediterranean diet lost a similar amount of weight but had better overall metabolic health and were more likely to stick with the plan. Long-term studies tracking people over many years also suggest that those who stick to the Mediterranean diet are less likely to become overweight or obese over time. People who have lost weight are less likely to regain it.

The Mediterranean diet doesn't cut out entire food groups, and it prioritizes real, unprocessed foods full of fiber and healthy fats. Unlike strict low-carb or high-protein plans, which can be hard to maintain, the Mediterranean approach is enjoyable and easy to integrate into daily life. Even without counting calories, many people find they naturally eat less and feel more satisfied. The modest portions of low glycemic index, fiber rich, unprocessed, wholegrain carbohydrate foods are key to optimize glucose regulation and insulin sensitivity. The proteins, often derived from plant sources such as beans are important for satiety and healthy fats such as those in olive oil and nuts reduce glycemic load. Bioactive compounds such as polyphenols in the colorful plant rich Mediterranean diet also have effects on insulin and glucose metabolism.

Importantly, some of its health benefits go beyond weight alone. Research shows that this diet can improve gut health and reduce harmful cholesterol even when calories aren't deliberately restricted. That means the quality of the food, not just the quantity, plays a key role in better health. Major health organizations now recommend the Mediterranean diet not only for heart health and diabetes prevention, but also as one of the best long-term strategies for healthy weight management.

Working with an Overweight Child

Childhood obesity remains a serious public health concern. The rates have risen sharply over the past few decades and remain high. According to the CDC, by 2017–2020, around 20 percent of US children aged six to 11 were living with obesity, a figure that has remained steady since the early 2000s but is still more than three times higher than in the 1980s. Obesity in childhood often persists into adulthood, without effective intervention, children with obesity have a 70 to 80 percent chance of becoming obese adults. That's why it's important to take action early, not through shame or blame, but with compassion, support, and practical steps.

The health impacts of obesity in children are significant. As well as increasing the risk of prediabetes and Type 2 diabetes, excess weight can cause joint pain, asthma, obstructive sleep apnea, high blood pressure, and liver dysfunction. Mental health is also affected. Many children with obesity experience bullying, low self-esteem, anxiety, and depression. Left unaddressed, some of these complications can appear as early as adolescence or young adulthood.

If you're a parent or caregiver of a child who is overweight or obese, here are some effective ways to support their health and well-being:

>> **Set a healthy example:** Children learn by observing, so one of the most powerful feats you can do is demonstrate healthy habits yourself. This includes preparing nutritious meals, enjoying regular movement, and creating a balanced relationship with food — not restrictive diets.

>> **Encourage daily physical activity:** All children need at least 60 minutes of moderate-to-vigorous physical activity per day. Encourage active play, limit screen time, and help your child find activities they enjoy — whether it's dancing, cycling, swimming, or walking the dog.

>> **Be aware of what they're eating:** Take an interest in your child's food environment at home and at school. Advocate for healthier school meals if needed and consider packing a balanced lunch if options are limited. Avoid using food as a reward and aim for structure in meal and snack times.

TIP

Focus on building lifelong healthy habits, not quick fixes. Support your child's confidence and self-worth, regardless of their weight, and involve them positively in changes — children do best when they feel empowered, not judged.

Chapter **10**

Living an Active Lifestyle

I f you don't exercise, you are missing out on the single most important, simplest, and least expensive tool for good health and long life that exists. Exercise can have a profound effect on prediabetes, diabetes, and the chance that prediabetes will proceed to diabetes. These are key long-term reasons to exercise. In the short term, exercise, especially vigorous exercise, promotes the secretion of pleasure hormones in your brain.

In this chapter, we explain the function of exercise both for your body and for your brain. We discuss how depression affects your willingness to exercise (or do anything else, for that matter) and how to fight against that inertia. We reveal how you likely got into the habit of not exercising and what you need to do to get out of it and make exercise a part of your daily life.

Why Exercise Is Essential for Optimal Human Function

Only during modern times have human beings lived sedentary lives. A sedentary lifestyle involves spending much of the day sitting, with limited physical activity. Prior to that, however, moving frequently was the only way that people could survive. Just like other mammals, our bodies are built for movement. While it's wonderful to enjoy the conveniences of cars, elevators, escalators, electric bikes, and so on, making sure that we move enough to stay healthy is now more important than ever.

Exercise is essential for humans of all ages. It boosts and maintains our mental, physical, and even spiritual health. According to the World Health Organization, "31% of adults and 80% of adolescents do not meet the recommended levels of physical activity." They report that the "global estimate of the cost of physical inactivity to public healthcare systems between 2020 and 2030 is about US $300 billion (approximately $27 billion per year) if levels of physical inactivity are not reduced."

Regular physical activity is widely recognized as one of the most effective ways to improve health and prevent disease, especially for people with prediabetes. Recent medical research strongly supports this.

For example, a 2025 review published in the journal *Frontiers in Endocrinology* found that both aerobic exercise (such as walking or cycling) and resistance training (such as weightlifting), as well as a combination of the two, significantly improved blood sugar control in people with prediabetes. The most effective approach for lowering fasting blood sugar was a combination of both types of exercise. Meanwhile, aerobic activity on its own was especially helpful for reducing blood sugar levels after meals and lowering HbA1c, the key marker of long-term blood sugar control.

The review also finds that the best results are seen in people who exercised at a moderate intensity for about 150–250 minutes per week. This exercise is roughly equivalent to 30–50 minutes a day, five days a week.

The American Diabetes Association (ADA), in its 2025 *Standards of Care*, also recommends regular physical activity for anyone at risk of diabetes, including those with prediabetes. According to the ADA, exercise not only helps regulate blood sugar, but also reduces the risk of heart disease and supports healthy weight management. Even moderate activities, such as brisk walking, can lead to big health improvements, and exercise plans should be personalized to suit each person's needs and abilities.

A 2024 study also published in *Frontiers in Endocrinology* that compared different types of exercise programs also finds that combining moderate-intensity aerobic activity with light to moderate resistance training led to the greatest improvements in blood sugar, body weight, and cholesterol levels for people with prediabetes.

One of the challenges with promoting exercise is that nowadays people have to make a conscious effort to do it. Prior to industrialization, when everything was done by hand, daily life itself was a workout. Nowadays, however, it isn't. People need time, energy, and motivation to exercise. One of the best ways to be inspired to exercise more is to ponder its many health benefits.

Here is just a short list of some of these benefits:

» Exercise prevents prediabetes from becoming diabetes.

» Exercise prevents *macrovascular disease:* the disease of any of the large blood vessels in the body. In other words, it prevents heart attacks, strokes, and *peripheral vascular disease* (the blockage of arteries that serve the legs).

» Exercise increases your self-esteem.

» Exercise reduces your risk of osteoporosis.

» Exercise reduces your risk of breast cancer.

» Exercise increases your strength and stamina.

» Exercise reduces depression (see the next section).

» Exercise diminishes the effect of stress (which we discuss in Chapter 9).

» Exercise can help you maintain weight loss or even cause weight loss if it's done for a sufficient amount of time.

» Exercise lowers your blood pressure.

» Exercise tones and firms your muscles.

» Exercise may help you to overcome substance abuse such as cigarette smoking and alcoholism.

» Exercise helps you sleep better.

» Exercise helps cognitive function.

» Exercise gives you more energy.

» Exercise helps improve mood.

» Exercise helps with mental illness.

» Exercise helps boost your metabolism and regulate hormones.

» Exercise helps you burn fat and build muscle.

» Exercise helps treat anxiety and depression.

In the following sections, we examine how some of these benefits work in detail.

Stopping prediabetes from becoming diabetes

If you're currently not very active and are thinking about starting an exercise routine, especially if you have prediabetes or other health concerns, talking to your healthcare provider first is a good idea. A medical check-up can help identify any limitations or risks, and your provider can recommend safe, effective ways to begin increasing your activity level. Starting gradually and choosing activities you enjoy can make it easier to build a lasting, healthy habit.

Numerous studies have shown that insulin action, fasting blood glucose levels, and glucose intolerance are all improved by exercise. One of the most important studies was published in *BMC Endocrine Disorders*. Sixteen men aged 19 to 23 did just seven and a half minutes of very high intensity exercise on a stationary bike per week for two weeks. That small amount of exercise led to a very significant improvement in their insulin sensitivity.

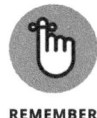

REMEMBER

If you are over 35 years old and have not exercised much before, you must visit your doctor for a consultation before you begin highly vigorous exercise.

Is it unrealistic for you to consider high intensity exercise? I don't think so. Start with ten-second "spurts" of activity with 30-second rests in between. Gradually build up to 30 seconds of high intensity with 30 seconds of rest between. Do that sequence five times in a row, and you are exercising at the same level as the people in the study.

A second important study (reported in *Applied Physiology, Nutrition, and Metabolism*) looked at the scientific evidence for the effect of exercise and concluded that "30 minutes per day of moderate- or high-level physical activity is an effective and safe way to prevent Type 2 diabetes in all populations."

So whether you want to go all out and get your exercise over with in 7½ minutes a week, or whether you want to work at a lower intensity and do 30 minutes a day, you can delay and perhaps prevent developing diabetes by exercising.

Preventing heart attacks, strokes, and peripheral vascular disease

The evidence that exercise can prevent macrovascular disease such as heart attacks, strokes, and peripheral vascular disease is just as strong. An article in the *Mayo Clinic Proceedings* in April 2009 made two important points on this subject:

>> Physical activity, exercise training, and overall cardiorespiratory fitness can prevent these diseases — the evidence is overwhelming.

>> For someone who already has cardiovascular disease, exercise can prevent it from recurring. (Unfortunately, patients don't use cardiovascular rehabilitation programs nearly often enough.)

Besides lowering your blood glucose, exercise prevents macrovascular disease by creating the following effects:

>> It lowers your blood pressure.

>> It lowers your total and bad cholesterol while raising your good cholesterol.

>> It lowers your stress levels.

These effects occur in all age groups, including the elderly and children. Bottom line: You are never too young or too old to exercise and benefit from it.

Increasing your self-esteem

From kids to adults, daily exercise reduces symptoms of depression and improves self-esteem. How do we know? In one study at the Medical College of Georgia, kids aged seven to 11 exercised for either 20 or 40 minutes each day after school for 13 weeks. Both groups of kids experienced improved self-esteem, but the 40-minute group benefited more than the 20-minute group. The kids did aerobic exercises such as running, jumping rope, and playing basketball and soccer.

Many studies show that older people experience the same esteem benefits from exercise. For example, a study from the Department of Psychology at Bishop's University asked 127 men and women to fill out questionnaires that assessed their self-esteem, body satisfaction, and body build. With both genders, people who exercised a lot reported higher self-esteem than people who didn't exercise much.

It doesn't seem to matter what kind of exercise you do. Increased self-esteem is a side effect whether you play a sport, do martial arts, do weight training, or run.

Reducing your risk of osteoporosis

Osteoporosis is a loss of bone tissue that occurs with age in both males and females and is exacerbated by the loss of the hormone estrogen when women hit menopause. If you lose too much bone, you can suffer from fractures in your hips and spine. Your doctor can determine your level of bone loss by doing a *bone densitometry study*: The lower the densitometry, the more bone you've lost.

Weight-bearing exercises seem to be best for preventing osteoporosis. *Weight-bearing* means that you exercise on your feet, with your bones supporting your weight. Dancing, using an elliptical training machine (which is easy on your joints), climbing stairs, gardening, and walking are examples of weight-bearing exercises. Swimming is not because the water, rather than your bones, is bearing your weight. Bike-riding is also not a weight-bearing exercise because you are sitting.

Other types of exercise, such as resistance exercise and flexibility exercise, are also necessary. When you do *resistance* exercise, you use your bones and muscles against the weight of some other object. *Flexibility* exercises improve your balance and prevent injuries. Some examples that you can choose from include:

>> Regular stretching

>> Tai Chi

>> Yoga

>> Pilates

I show you some specific resistance exercises and offer some advice about stretching in Chapter 17.

Maintaining or increasing your weight loss

If you've already lost weight, you can maintain that loss with exercise. But it takes a bit more exercise to actually lose more weight. The key in both situations is to do some moderate-intensity exercise for a long enough time.

You find the best information concerning how much exercise you need to maintain weight loss in the National Weight Control Registry (www.nwcr.ws). Begun in 1994, it has been following thousands of people who have maintained at least a 30-pound weight loss for one year or longer. Members have lost an average of 66 pounds and kept the weight off for five and a half years. Here are just a few stats gleaned from this registry:

>> Loss of weight has been as low as 30 pounds and as high as 300 pounds.

>> Those who lost weight have kept it off from one year to 66 years.

>> Those who have lost weight rapidly or taken as long as 14 years to lose their weight.

>> Walking is the most frequent form of physical activity for the registry members.

>> Most members follow a low-fat, reduced-calorie diet.

>> 90 percent of members exercise, on average, one hour per day.

What if you want to lose more pounds? The American College of Sports Medicine recommends at least 250 minutes of moderately vigorous exercise a week to lose weight. With that much exercise and just a small reduction in daily kilocalories (say 200 kilocalories), you can lose about a pound a week. In three months, you will lose 12 pounds. Even without reducing your food intake at all, you may lose two pounds in three weeks.

Examples of moderate-intensity exercise are:

>> Walking two miles in 30 minutes

>> Playing doubles tennis

>> Dancing rapidly

>> Jogging one mile in 14 minutes

>> Swimming slowly

THE DYNAMICS OF EXERCISE

Exercise increases your body's demand for both glucose and fat for energy. The glucose leaves your liver and the fat leaves your fat tissue, and they both go to your muscles. Here's how these processes happen when you exercise:

• The storage form of glucose in the liver (called *glycogen*) breaks down and releases its glucose. After the glycogen is used up by continued exercise, your liver can make large amounts of glucose from *amino acids,* the building blocks of protein.

• If you exercise at a steady and moderate pace, your glucose production decreases and your body turns to fat for energy.

• If you exercise very vigorously, your liver produces more glucose. Sometimes the glucose production outpaces the use of the glucose by your muscles, and your blood glucose rises for a while. Vigorous exercise usually doesn't last very long, and the extra glucose replenishes your muscles when the exercise ends.

Bottom line: Glucose is your energy source when you exercise vigorously, and fat is your energy source during less intense exercise. To lose fat, focus on steady, moderate exercise.

You don't have to put in as much time if you do vigorous exercise. You need to find out for yourself how much time is necessary for weight loss, depending on how vigorously you exercise. Examples of vigorous exercise are:

>> Jogging one mile in 12 minutes

>> Playing singles tennis, squash, or racquetball

>> Running 10-minute miles

>> Dancing vigorously

>> Skiing downhill or cross country

>> Rowing, canoeing, or kayaking vigorously

>> Bicycling at 10 to 16 miles per hour

Using Exercise to Combat Depression

Exercise and fresh air have both been linked to improving mood and helping people with depression. People get depressed for many reasons. Sometimes the depression is an appropriate response, such as when you lose a loved one, a home, or a job. Other times, depression can be a result of a hormonal imbalance or medical concern. But sometimes you feel depressed and don't understand why.

For someone with a health condition such as prediabetes, depression is especially problematic because you simply can't take optimal care of yourself when you're depressed. You're much more likely to make poor food choices, overeat, and exacerbate your health problems when you're struggling with depression.

Medications and psychotherapy may help, but exercise should be part of any plan to combat depression. In this section, we explain why.

Inactivity contributes to depression

Confession time: Doctors don't know everything. One detail we don't know is exactly how lack of exercise contributes to depression. However, we have some theories, including these:

>> **Exercise raises the level of *neurotransmitters* in your brain:** the chemicals that permit your brainwaves to move. This increase tends to improve your mood. Without activity, these chemicals are not secreted.

>> **Exercise raises your levels of *endorphins*:** chemicals that are like physiological opium. Endorphins help you to sleep better, decrease tension in your muscles, and decrease the production of stress hormones like cortisol in your body.

>> **Exercise raises your body temperature slightly,** which may have a calming effect.

Lower levels of neurotransmitters and endorphins may lead to anger, anxiety, fatigue, sadness, and many other symptoms associated with depression.

Depression contributes to inactivity

When you are depressed for any reason, you tend to lose interest in yourself and your environment. You develop an "I don't care" kind of attitude. Under these circumstances, you are not interested in being careful about what you eat, taking your medications, and doing exercise.

This situation qualifies as a Catch-22: a no-win situation. (The concept comes from the novel *Catch-22* by Joseph Heller. One of the novel's characters is an airman who is crazy and should not be allowed to fly missions during World War II. But if he asks to be grounded, that action would be considered sane, and therefore he'd be allowed to fly.) You're depressed and don't want to exercise. And because you don't exercise, your depression doesn't improve.

If you don't find a way to break out of this no-win situation, you'll likely continue to struggle with depression. For specific ideas of how to break the cycle, read the next section.

Planning to Move

So what steps do you have to take to start a successful exercise regimen. Here are some suggestions:

>> **Start with a realistic goal:** For example, in four months I want to be able to jog for 30 minutes. Or in three months I want to be able to lift 60 pounds over my head 18 times.

>> **Examine your obstacles:** If you have physical limitations, you need to start with a type of exercise that works for you. Time constraints? Consider exercising in short intervals. New to exercise? Start very slowly — even a few minutes a day.

>> **Break the goal down into small improvements:** For example, each day I want to add 15 seconds to the duration of my jogging. Each week I want to add five pounds to the weights that I lift over my head.

>> **Gather the equipment you need:** It may include a set of weights, a stop-watch, or even a GPS training watch. This wonderful device, made by many manufacturers (including Garmin, Timex, and others) enables you to:

- Measure the time of exercise

- Measure the distance of exercise

- Measure the speed of exercise and change it "on the run"

TIP

You can alter your workout easily by adding time, adding distance, going faster, or combining any of those changes.

>> **Consider starting with a personal trainer:** These highly trained individuals can make sure that you are doing your exercise properly from the beginning. You're much better off learning the right way to exercise at first — otherwise, you have to unlearn the wrong way. Explain to your trainer that you are not in a hurry; you want to build up gradually, but you have a definite goal.

Start slowly If you're out of shape, or are new to exercise, you don't have to go crazy on the first day, even five minutes of exercise is better than nothing. Add a simple minute a day until you build yourself up to your goal.

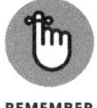

REMEMBER

You don't have to like exercise to reap its benefits. Jack Lalanne, also known as the "Godfather of Fitness" who was a fitness and nutritional expert and world leader in the health and fitness movement who lived to be 96 years old, repeatedly stated that he hated working out, yet he did it for over two hours each morning and inspired people worldwide to be happier and healthier.

Of course, it's our hope that you pick a physical activity that you enjoy, and that you grow even more fond of it once you note how it makes you feel. But even if you don't that's okay. Just start from where you are knowing that you are doing good for your mind and body.

Exercising through your depression

As we discuss earlier, you find many different reasons for depression and it's a complex topic that effects people differently. Seeking out professional treatment is important if you or a loved one displays symptoms of clinical depression. In addition to the proper protocol, laughing, exercise, and spending time outdoors can be part of an effective treatment plan.

Laughing, and hearing others laugh, is known to improve the mood. Try making yourself laugh even if you don't have anything to laugh about. Just perform the physical act of laughing. As you continue to laugh, suddenly, you can begin to feel happier. You are performing the end result of amusement, and you start to feel amused. This action is essentially what happens when you listen to a good comedian. He starts you laughing (presumably by saying something really funny), and after a while, everything is funny. Some doctors even prescribe laugh therapy to patients by recommending that they listen to people laughing on YouTube videos.

You can accomplish the same thing with exercise and fresh air. Start walking and spending time outdoors if possible, for just a few minutes a day. The feeling that you can actually do something will begin to alter your perception that you can't do anything. Your perception will change even more if you continue to add seconds and prolong your exercise each day. You may still need a psychologist and medications to help you, but you also may find that as you do more and more exercise, you can leave those other tools behind.

Finding time

The best way to overcome this roadblock to exercise is to examine how you spend your time each day. For one day, write down what you do every minute, starting the moment you wake up. Here's an example:

- » 6:15: Awake
- » 6:15-6:30: Bathroom
- » 6:30-7:00: Journaling and meditation
- » 7:00-8:24: Breakfast
- » 8:24-9:15: Responded to emails and calls
- » 9:15-10:00 Showered, groomed, and dressed
- » 10:00-12:30: Online meetings
- » 12:30-1:15: Lunch
- » 1:15-5:00: Wrote *Prediabetes For Dummies* plus bathroom
- » 5:00-5:30: Exercised on the elliptical trainer
- » 5:30-6:15: Showered, groomed, and dressed
- » 6:15-7:15: Social media
- » 7:15-8:00: Dinner with friends
- » 8:00-9:00: Went for a stroll outside

>> 9:00-10:00: Read

>> 10:00-10:30: Meditation

>> 10:30 p.m.-6:00 a.m: Sleep

When you truly track what you do, it becomes easier to make adjustments and to make more of your time. It also becomes easier to eliminate distractions and transform them.

Try doing the same time study for yourself. You may be amazed by how much time you can find to do a little more exercise. We always find it curious that the busiest people we know seem to have the most time to do what they need to do.

What if your time study reveals that the only way to exercise is to sleep even less than you already do? If you simply can't do 30 minutes of exercise each day, start by making time to do two and a half minutes of high intensity exercise every day. Just that small amount can make a huge difference in your health, both physically and mentally.

Turning off your TV or computer

You need to set screen-time boundaries, not just for your children but for yourself. Outside of your work hours, limit yourself to a maximum of two hours of screen time a day (including TV, computer monitors, cell phones, and GPS devices).

If you can't accomplish this goal on your own, get a device called the TV Allowance (www.tvallowance.com). Set it for yourself, as well as for your kids. And don't forget that your kids tend to do as you do, not as you say. Use your newly found extra time to demonstrate to your kids the importance of exercising, reading, preparing healthy meals, and so on.

REMEMBER

You *do* have enough time, enough energy, and enough motivation to exercise. You don't have to strive to become a world-class athlete — just to do enough exercise to prevent going from prediabetes to diabetes and to move back from prediabetes to a healthy state.

Chapter **11**

Managing Stress and Seeking Joy

You can't avoid stress. You likely experience it in your job, in your family, in your relationships, in the world around you, and within yourself. And stress can make you sick if it causes you to stop eating properly, maintaining your hygiene, taking necessary medications, protecting yourself against contagious disease, and exercising.

In this chapter, we point out possible sources of stress in your life — both those you can change and those you can't. We discuss how stress affects your food intake and may contribute to prediabetes. We offer suggestions for not only minimizing the impact of stress in your life, but also for finding your joy, which is the best antidote to stress. And finally, we discuss the special situations of stress for the elderly and for kids.

Adopting a Healthy Mentality around Stress and Joy

"Necessity is the mother of invention" is often said, which is especially true when it comes to stress. When not managed properly, stress can lead to chronic health problems, but when it is transformed, it can actually help us to achieve our goals. The next time you feel stressed, think about what is underneath the "stressful" feeling. Whether you're worried about meeting a work deadline, missing a plane, or something out of your control, the stress that you're perceiving is telling you what really matters.

The next time you're stressed, thank the stress for pointing out to you what you really want. It may seem awkward in the beginning, but the act of imagining takes your mind off of what you don't want and helps you focus on what you actually like. If you're worried about missing a deadline, you may be worried about losing your job or losing credibility or appearing to be incompetent. After you identify which fear you have, you can shift your attention to enjoying wonderful sense of job security, being respected by your peers, and loving your work or the income that your work provides. Focusing on what feels good is good for you.

DR. POOLE'S STRESS MANAGEMENT PRINCIPLES

When discussing stress with his patients, Dr. Poole developed the following principles. A psychologically healthy response to stress involves:

- Recognizing that we can control only our own actions and thoughts, not other people or external conditions

- Focusing on what is within our control — our perceptions, choices, and problem-solving efforts

- Taking personal responsibility for our reactions rather than blaming circumstances or others

- Using internal motivation to make choices that align with our needs in constructive ways (for example, seeking connection rather than withdrawal when stressed)

Learning the technique of pivoting (redirecting your thoughts from negative ones to positive ones) can help adopt a healthy attitude toward stress. It can also cause a shift in mentality that enables you not only to protect your health but also to perceive solutions to the challenges that you're facing. Remember back to the last time that you were stressed out. Did you ever come up with a solution by dwelling on the problem and feeling "stuck"? Most times the so-called solutions come when we're washing the dishes, taking a shower, going for a walk, or basically, doing other activities — even busy work or mundane task.

The next time you feel truly stuck, try doing one of these actions:

>> Thinking about a happy memory and dwelling on it

>> Going for a walk

>> Stretching

>> Watch a comedy

>> Listen to beautiful music

>> Sing

>> Dance

>> Take three deep breaths in and out

After doing one or all these actions, try saying to yourself "I don't know how to _____, but the universe does." Admitting that you don't know the answer, but the universe does helps to take the stress off of you. Try to adopt the notion that there really is a solution, that you are worthy of having it, and allowing it to show itself to you.

After you do this, try to distract yourself with something joyful. Joy is the perfect antidote for stress and the more joy you feel the less stress you will be.

Considering What Brings You the Most Joy

Practicing your favorite activity, talking and socializing with those you love, hugging a friend, or listening to nature can all reduce your stress levels if they bring you joy. If you value good health, your daily goal should be to attempt to be as happy as possible, to spend as little time as possible focusing on problems. When you engage in practices that make you happy — no matter what they are, stress (at least during that time) is eradicated. Joy is the highest positive emotion on the emotional scale, and when you're feeling it, you can't simultaneously feel stressed.

As simple as it sounds, finding time for joy, fun, happiness, and even relaxation is a luxury for many people. Modern societies often portray those emotions as frivolous and tend to place more worth or importance on busy people who are stressed with their very important activities. But maintaining this mentality and living a lifestyle in accordance with it will only result in increased inflammation, irregular blood glucose levels, and many other health complications, in addition to an increased risk of depression and anxiety.

Prioritizing your happiness

For the sake of your own health, dedicating as much time as you can doing what you love is in your best interest. Any activities that allow you to "lose yourself" while taking part in them — whether it's cooking or golf or dancing or reading — are the perfect way to keep stress at bay.

Of course, if you tell people about this, they may respond with "I wish I had time to do that" or "it must be nice to have so much free time!" They may attempt to make you feel guilty, or as if you're not as committed to other areas of your life because you do those joyful activities. If this happens, that's okay. Let them say these things. Or don't share what you're doing with people whom you feel won't understand.

The truth of the matter is that everyone has 24 hours each day to make choices. Of course responsibilities and other external factors may influence your schedule heavily, but if you analyze your schedule closely, you can find a way to replace some "down time" or even other times with activities you love.

Finding time to do what brings you joy

When scheduling fun into your calendar, take into account a few details:

>> Which activities do you enjoy most, and are there specific times that they need to be done? For example, most outdoor sports and activities are done during the day. You can go to the gym anytime you like. Reading doesn't have a time limit, but organized group activities do.

>> Write down the times that the activities you like to do can be done.

>> Take a look at your actual schedule — including accurate travel times, errands, socializing, and so forth and try scheduling an additional fun event into your schedule each week.

>> After you're comfortable with the additional item, switch to two activities, and then three, and so on until you're fitting in as much fun as possible.

>> If there's anything on your schedule that you can let go of or delegate, do so. That way you have more time for what you enjoy.

>> Get friends and family involved in the activities that you like — this way you have accountability partners.

Recognizing Sources of Stress in Your Life

Feelings of stress are normal. Your body responds to various threats (both physical and psychological) with a fight-or-flight reaction. The result is the production of hormones such as adrenaline and cortisol, both of which raise your blood glucose to provide more fuel for your muscles and brain. These hormones have side effects, which make you aware that you are under stress. What are some of the side effects?

>> Your hearts pounds.

>> Your chest muscles contract, and you have trouble breathing.

>> You *hyperventilate,* which means you breathe too rapidly and feel light-headed.

>> Your arms and legs become shaky.

>> Your throat feels tense.

>> You clench your jaw.

When you're under stress, you may develop one or more symptoms, which are divided into four major categories: physical, emotional, behavioral, and cognitive. Here are some of the biggies:

>> Physical symptoms
- Aches and pains
- Diarrhea or constipation
- Frequent colds
- Loss of sex drive

>> Emotional symptoms
- Depression
- Feeling overwhelmed
- Irritability
- Moodiness

» Behavioral symptoms

  ● Isolating yourself

  ● Eating too much or too little

  ● Developing nervous habits, such as nail biting

  ● Neglecting responsibilities

» Cognitive (thinking) symptoms

  ● Anxious thoughts

  ● Constant worrying

  ● Inability to concentrate

  ● Poor judgment

You can see what a profound effect stress can have on your health. We say more about that connection later in this chapter.

Categories of stress

You should be aware of different kinds of stress:

» *Acute stress* results from a recent situation or problem or a problem you anticipate in the near future. For example, an auto accident, a deadline for a report, or a robbery can cause acute stress. Because the stressors are short-term, this type of stress isn't as damaging as other kinds. You may have symptoms such as a pounding heart, dizziness, or headaches, but they subside as the acute stress subsides.

» *Episodic acute stress* occurs in people who live very disorganized lives. These people are overburdened with responsibilities that they can't manage. They are highly competitive, hostile, and insecure, and they have constant head-aches, chest pain, and gastrointestinal symptoms such as diarrhea. Treating episodic acute stress is much more difficult than treating acute stress because the disorganized lifestyle is so ingrained in the individual. People in this situation often need long-term professional help.

» *Chronic stress* results from situations that go on and on, such as the situation in the Middle East between Arabs and Jews or a long-term, unhappy marriage. People with chronic stress feel trapped and may give up trying to solve the problem. Often they go on living their lives hopelessly and die of a heart attack or suicide. These people are the most difficult to treat because they feel certain that they are "stuck."

Stressors can be further divided into those you can change and those that are out of your control. Some of the stressors may seem like happy events to you (such as an engagement, a new baby, a new house, or a new job), but they are still sources of stress.

Stressors you can change

You may like to believe that you have control over just about everything but some situations are easier to change than others. That said, the process of changing any source of stress in your life often causes additional stress! Your task is to determine if the increase in short-term stress will result in a decrease in stress in the long haul. For example,

>> If you're engaged but not certain that the marriage will be right for you, you may be better off breaking the engagement.

>> If you're in a very stressful marriage, divorce (despite the stress it creates) may ultimately be your best choice.

>> If you have ongoing problems with a friend, a neighbor, or a relative, you may need to take action that is difficult in the short term but will pay off by reducing your stress later.

>> If you're in a financial mess, you likely need to make some tough choices now (such as taking a second job or cutting out any unessential expenses) that will reduce your long-term stress.

>> If you've got legal problems, you're probably better off facing any tough consequences now rather than trying to delay them. The stress will only increase with each day that your situation remains in limbo.

Stressors out of your control

Many stressors fall into this category because they're created by other people or events that you can't control. Some common examples of stress outside your control include:

>> Buying or selling a home (because of a work relocation, for example)

>> Separating from a loved one

>> Getting a divorce

>> Losing your job and starting a new one

>> Retiring (even if you've been looking forward to it)

- » Getting emotionally or physically ill

- » Watching a spouse, family member, or friend go through a bad illness

- » Experiencing the death of a spouse, family member, or friend

- » Getting pregnant and giving birth

Unforeseen catastrophes and misfortune

TIP

For a much more extensive list of stressors, check out `http://stresscourse.tripod.com/id14.html`. At this site, you can find a checklist called "Cooper's Life Stress Inventory." You check off the stressors in your life and select the severity of the stress from 1 (low level) to 10 (very severe). You add up the numbers and grade yourself. If you score 100 or more, you are under high stress. If this is the case, you may want to seek out a coach, counselor, therapist, or other type of guide to help your particular situation and to talk to.

Assessing Your Attitude toward Your Stressors

How you perform under stress is greatly affected by your personality. Each of us has a set of personality traits, many of which are similar to other people's traits. These sets of traits categorize us as *Type A* or *Type B* personalities. Many people have traits that fall in both sets, but most of us have traits that predominate in one group or the other. Table 11-1 shows how Type A and Type B personalities differ.

TABLE 11-1   **Type A and Type B Personality Traits**

Type A Traits	Type B Traits
Always in a hurry	Never in a hurry
Can't quietly listen	Listens until the other person is finished
Doesn't like to wait	Waits calmly
Excessively competitive	Not excessively competitive
Holds feelings in	Can express feelings
Must finish things	Can leave things unfinished

Type A Traits	Type B Traits
Never late	Unhurried about appointments
Minimal social activities	Many social activities
Tries to do several activities	Does one activity at a time
Wants everything perfect	Can accept imperfection

Looking carefully at yourself

As you look at Table 11-1, you may find it relatively easy to see where you fit in. The traits on the left are tight and tense. If you see yourself on that side of the table, you are subject to high stress. Events in your life trigger stress reactions that are not good for your health. You are subject to the signs and symptoms of stress that we list earlier in the chapter. You may also be depressed, feel overwhelmed, overeat, or worry constantly.

If you identify more with the right side of the table, you are probably pretty laid back. When stressors come along, you take a more philosophical attitude. You think more in terms of "This too shall pass." You are much less likely to be made sick by stress than someone with a Type A personality.

Of course, many people are in denial. They can't see themselves clearly. You may want to ask others (especially a spouse) to provide some input about which side of the table you fit in. But generally speaking, if you feel constantly under pressure, you're very likely a Type A personality.

Giving yourself a break

If you're a Type A personality, you may be setting yourself up for sickness. When you react with a fight-or-flight response, you are using an ancient coping behavior that's often not useful for modern sources of stress. Sure, if the stress is a car that is about to hit you, the flight response is exactly what you need. Those types of circumstances are rare, however. Most of the stressors we list in this chapter require you to think calmly about the problem and solve it if possible.

The way we think about the stress plays a major role in our ability to handle it. Back in 1917, Italian playwright Luigi Pirandello (who won the Nobel Prize for Literature in 1934) had the first performance of his play *It Is So (If You Think So)*. He went on to write a number of plays with the same theme, which is this:

> The way we think things are determines our reaction to them, whether our observation of things is true or not!

Pirandello wasn't the first person to write on this theme. It goes back to the ancient Greeks, but Pirandello's plays made it explicit. Characters in his plays are constantly misinterpreting what they observe and damaging themselves or others by their reactions.

Take the example of losing a job. For one person it may be a highly stressful event that provokes worries about finances and the ability to take care of their family, undermines their self-esteem, and so forth. For another, the same event may represent a chance to stop doing something that they found uninteresting or tedious or something that didn't pay enough. The second person may have the perspective that they now have an opportunity to take a break and rethink their career. The take-home message is that how you think about a situation determines whether you respond with a smile or with sickness.

What personality traits are most helpful in meeting the stresses that come our way? Dr. Susan Kobasa studied executives at the Bell Telephone Company while it was being restructured in the late 1970s and observed that three important personality traits were present in executives who did not respond to the stress with sickness. They were:

>> **Commitment:** Committed people are involved in their families, their work, and their communities. This commitment motivates them to work harder and gives them a purpose.

>> **Control:** People have one of two traits when it comes to control:

- An *internal locus of control,* which means you believe you have some influence on external events

- An *external locus of control,* which means you think you are simply an observer in life, and everything that happens to you is due to destiny

Obviously, people with an internal locus of control believe that they can do something about a stressor, which is healthier than the alternative.

>> **Challenge:** This term refers to the way you see the stressor. Do you see it as something to be overcome or as something that will overcome you? People who can deal with a challenge accept that change is inevitable. They welcome change as a chance to learn something new.

REMEMBER

These three traits — commitment, control, and challenge — are not necessarily built in to your DNA. They are *learned,* and everyone — including you — can learn or unlearn them. So give yourself a break, and learn how to cope with stress without getting sick.

Linking Your Stress Level to Your Relationship with Food

People under stress tend to consume foods that aren't good for their health. They eat fast foods, drink a lot of caffeine, eat foods that are high in fats and refined carbohydrates, and drink alcohol. People are especially susceptible during the holiday season, when lack of time, lack of money, and the pressure to give gifts are major stressors. In Chapter 9, we discuss the negative effects of eating that kind of diet over a long period of time.

Studies at the University of California–San Francisco have shown that one normal response to the secretion of stress hormones (especially cortisol) is to search for pleasurable food such as chocolate, pastries, and other sweets. These foods are called "comfort foods" for a good reason.

The logical explanation for all these research results is that sweet foods give us the glucose that we need for the fight-or-flight response. However, other circumstances are going on. One is that most of us are taught as children that we get a treat in response to sadness or physical discomfort. (Maybe your mother would give you a cookie after she cleaned off your scraped knee.) In addition, when we're stressed, we pay less attention to what we're putting in our mouths. Stress also causes us to drink a little extra alcohol to dampen the pain.

Finally, stress — particularly chronic stress — causes a number of symptoms and even diseases that result in problems with food. It forces an alteration in diet that may not be helpful to the person with prediabetes. Among the medical symptoms and diseases that stress can provoke are:

>> Colitis: An inflammatory disease of the large intestine

>> Gastritis: Inflammation of the stomach

>> Irritable bowel syndrome: Cramping, abdominal pain, bloating, constipation, or diarrhea that does not permanently harm the intestine

>> Obesity

>> Stomach and duodenal ulcers

>> Stomach pain

Avoiding Exercise Because of Stress

Just as we tend to eat too much of the wrong kinds of foods in a stressful situation, we also tend to stop exercising. A survey by the American Psychological Association showed that people under stress tend to discontinue their exercise program. They turn to sedentary behaviors such as watching TV, sleeping, overeating, and drinking to manage their stress, especially during the holidays.

REMEMBER

Stopping exercise is exactly the wrong reaction to stress because exercise is such an important part of reducing stress. We discuss your body's need for exercise (especially during stressful times) in depth in Chapter 10.

Realizing How Stress Contributes to Prediabetes

By now, you should have a pretty clear sense of how stress contributes to prediabetes. Stress causes us to do many of the things that predispose us to prediabetes and to stop doing things that prevent it. In response to stress, we tend to:

>> Stop exercising

>> Stop eating carefully

>> Use poor judgment

>> Avoid contact with people who could help us

>> Believe that we have no control over our lives and stop trying

When all these negative behaviors are taking place, the chances of you developing prediabetes (and diabetes) increase significantly.

Understanding Stress in the Elderly

The elderly are subject to sources of stress that are different from children and younger adults. Here are some of the most frequent sources of stress in the elderly:

>> Declining health

>> Decreased strength, mental ability, and balance

- » Reduced income

- » The sickness or death of a spouse

- » The sickness or death of other relatives and friends

- » Fear of an attack at home

- » Social isolation (as friends and relatives die)

All these stressors, and many others, can easily lead to end results such as poor eating habits, lack of exercise, and other physical behaviors that are extremely detrimental. That's one reason that this age group has the largest number of people with prediabetes and diabetes.

If you recognize yourself (or a loved one) in the description we're offering here, you can take a number of steps to reduce the stresses that seem inevitable for the elderly:

- » **Get involved in group activities:** Socializing with other people the same age can help you learn about solutions that others have discovered. If nothing else, it gives you the opportunity to vent to people who understand what you're experiencing.

- » **Take time to relax and rest your body:** At the same time, don't stop doing exercise because it can help so much to reduce stress.

- » **Be extremely careful about what and how much you eat:** Your metabolism is likely slower than it used to be, which means you may gain weight easily.

- » **Avoid cigarettes and alcohol**

- » **Get enough sleep**

- » **Learn something new:** Start to do something you've always wanted to do but never had enough time for, such as playing the piano or speaking a new language.

In a study published in *Adultspan Journal*, elderly people living in nursing homes were questioned about how they cope with stress. They mentioned the following three methods most often:

- » Praying

- » Reading, watching TV, or listening to music

- » Talking to friends and family

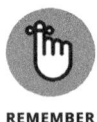

While nothing is wrong with any of these methods, focusing on healthy food and exercise need to be high on the list of coping mechanisms as well.

Perceiving Stress in Kids

Unfortunately, young people aren't immune to stress. Even though they don't have to pay bills or hold down jobs, kids have their own stressors that are as significant for them as adult stressors are for you. The following sections describe common stresses for kids and how to reduce them.

Identifying sources of stress

Kids have plenty of stresses. The stresses can be external (such as the expectations of parents) or internal (such as their desire to fit in socially). Some of their major stressors include:

>> Separation from parents when they have to go to preschool or school

>> Pressures of school and social activities

>> Pressure from having to keep up with too many activities, including schoolwork, athletics, and music lessons

>> Sympathetic stress from hearing the troubles of their parents

>> Sympathetic stress from learning about world problems (such as poverty or disease)

>> Divorce or other family problems

Reducing stress

Kids need the help of adults to reduce their stress because they may not see a way out on their own. Here are some of the ways you can help them:

>> **Listen without Judgment:** Offer a sympathetic ear and make children feel comfortable telling you the truth, even though they are scared of the consequences. Sometimes just being heard is enough to reduce stress substantially.

>> **Reduce the schedule:** If your child is overscheduled, suggest eliminating some activities. Too many scheduled activities can cause anxiety and depression in children.

- >> **Be honest but reassuring:** Don't try to sugarcoat or minimize divorce, financial problems, or other family issues. Chances are your child already knows how severe the problem is, so discuss it openly with them. That said, there is a big difference between making children aware of problems and involving them in the daily drama surrounding it. Children shouldn't be put in the middle of their parents' problems or be involved in all the financial problems and family issues. They need to constantly be reminded that whatever stressful situation is taking place that it's not their fault and that they are loved. By teaching kids that "everything will be okay" they learn at a young age how to face challenges and overcome obstacles.

- >> **Offer perspective:** Put world problems into perspective for your child. For example, the world economy may be bad, but your own family is doing fine. Offer them the opportunity to speak with a therapist if they need it.

- >> **Reduce screen time:** Free up time for homework, outside activities, and exercise by getting your kids away from the TV and computer.

- >> **Think like a child:** Anticipate and prepare your kids for activities that they find stressful, such as dentist's appointments.

Planning for Play Time

Just as adults need to make time for joy, so do kids. Children benefit a great deal from play times. Help your child identify types of activities where they can get fresh air, physical activity and socialize. Of course, each kid is different, some may like group sports, others quiet walks in the woods. Whatever healthy activities they enjoy, make sure that they get time to do it.

If other members of the family enjoy the same types of activities as the children do, doing them together is great. Cognitive, physical, social, and emotional development are all improved in children who enjoy adequate play time.

REMEMBER

Noting that creative play time and screen time are not the same is important, even though they often get mistaken for each other nowadays.

Obstacle courses, treasure hunting and hide and seek, local playgrounds, writing, painting, craft-making, coloring, cooking, baking, and sports are all examples of playtime activities for kids. Treat your kids to the very personal favor of helping them find the playtime that they need and love.

4

The Benefits of Following the Mediterranean Diet

Chapter **12**

Defining the Mediterranean Diet and How It Can Help

I f you or someone you care about has recently been diagnosed with prediabetes, you may worry that your future has to involve a lifetime of bland, uninspired meals. The truth, however, is far more encouraging, and if you follow the advice in this book, having been diagnosed with prediabetes may actually mean you can learn how to enjoy a far healthier and satisfying lifestyle.

The Mediterranean diet is one of the most effective ways to improve blood sugar, support a healthy weight, and lower the risk of heart disease is not just healthy — it's also delicious.

The Mediterranean diet is a joyful, time-tested way of eating focusing on colorful vegetables, fruits, whole grains, beans, nuts, seeds, extra virgin olive oil, fish, and modest portions of dairy and poultry. Meals are typically simple and without the unnecessary added ingredients of ultra-processed foods, bursting with flavor from the freshest seasonal ingredients, and often enjoyed in the company of family or friends. Rather than being a restrictive, short-term "diet," the Mediterranean approach is a flexible and sustainable pattern you can shape to your own tastes, local foods, and cultural traditions.

Year after year, the Mediterranean diet stands out as the "Best Overall Diet," according to expert panels such as those at *U.S. News & World Report*, based on its exceptional balance, nutritional completeness, and proven benefits for health and disease prevention. It also achieves the best results for heart health, prediabetes and diabetes control, and stands apart from fad diets by being practical, enjoyable, and backed by decades of reliable research.

For people with prediabetes, the Mediterranean diet is especially powerful: it emphasizes high-fiber, low-glycemic foods that help steady blood sugar levels, and it features healthy fats from extra virgin olive oil and nuts, which can improve your body's response to insulin. Perhaps most importantly, this is an eating style you'll want to stick with — not just for its health rewards for many chronic conditions including those associated with prediabetes, but also for the sheer satisfaction of good food, shared with others, over the course of a full and healthy life.

In this chapter you discover more about the Mediterranean diet and how it works for prediabetes.

Understanding the Mediterranean Diet

The Mediterranean diet is built from many common food types, with a balance of healthy macronutrients, micronutrients and bioactive compounds which are explored later in this chapter. However, it's not just a list of foods, but a way of eating that has grown and changed over centuries. It is built around a wide range of plant foods such as colorful and varied vegetables, leafy greens, fruit, beans, lentils, nuts, and seeds, along with whole grains such as barley and farro. Extra virgin olive oil is the main source of fat, used for cooking and dressing foods. Fish and other seafood appear regularly, while meat and dairy are eaten in smaller amounts. Ultra-processed foods are completely absent. This way of eating reflects the produce and seafood available locally, but it has also been shaped by trade and cultural exchange. Foods we now think of as central, such as tomatoes, coffee, and some spices, were introduced from other parts of the world, while dark chocolate arrived from the Americas and became part of the region's food culture.

You find no single version of the Mediterranean diet. The ingredients and dishes vary from place to place. The foods in a Sicilian market differ from those in a Greek fishing village or a Moroccan town, but the principles are similar: meals are based on fresh, seasonal ingredients and prepared in ways that bring out their natural flavor. Many traditional dishes balance flavors such as the slight bitterness of olives or leafy greens with the sharpness of garlic and herbs, or the warmth of spices such as cinnamon and cumin. The result is food that is straightforward, satisfying, and connected to the land and history of the region.

Looking at the Mediterranean Diet Pyramid

For a visual depiction of the Mediterranean diet, it's possible to find a number of images that illustrate the most common foods in a typical Mediterranean-style eating pattern. A pyramid is often used because it makes it easy to show the foundation of the diet with foods eaten daily in generous amounts occupying the broad base, with those enjoyed less frequently appearing higher up in smaller sections. At the base you typically see vegetables, fruits, whole grains, legumes, nuts, seeds, herbs, spices, and extra virgin olive oil, followed by fish and seafood, then poultry, eggs, and dairy in moderate amounts, and finally red meat and sweets at the narrow top, to be consumed only occasionally.

The concept of the Mediterranean Diet Pyramid (see Figure 12-1) was first formally developed in 1993 by the non-profit Oldways Preservation and Exchange Trust, in partnership with the Harvard School of Public Health and the World Health Organization. It was designed as a simple, culturally authentic guide to the eating patterns traditionally found in Mediterranean countries in the mid-20th century, when rates of chronic disease were among the lowest in the world and life expectancy among the highest.

Since then, other organizations have refined and adapted the concept, creating updated versions to reflect new scientific evidence and the diversity of Mediterranean food cultures. These include the Mediterranean Diet Foundation in Spain, which has developed a pyramid emphasizing fresh, local, and seasonal produce, and the UNESCO recognition of the Mediterranean diet as an "Intangible Cultural Heritage of Humanity," highlighting not only the foods themselves but also the social and cultural traditions of shared meals. While the details of these pyramids may differ slightly, they all promote the same core principles: an abundance of plant-based foods, healthy fats, especially extra virgin olive oil, moderate portions of animal products, and a focus on pleasure and sustainability in eating.

TIP

Many traditional versions of the Mediterranean Diet Pyramid include moderate wine consumption, typically red wine with meals, as part of the cultural and culinary tradition. However, in recent years there's been growing caution about including any alcohol, as even low levels are now known to elevate the risk of certain cancers. Simultaneously, researchers from the landmark PREDIMED Mediterranean diet trial, focusing on older adults, have cautioned that excluding wine from the Mediterranean eating pattern may reduce the diet's protective effects by up to around 23 percent, according to their interpretation. Ongoing studies are exploring whether drinking a modest amount of wine in the Mediterranean manner, always with meals and specifically with the other foods of the diet, may mitigate harms or retain health benefits, but the findings remain preliminary and should be interpreted with care.

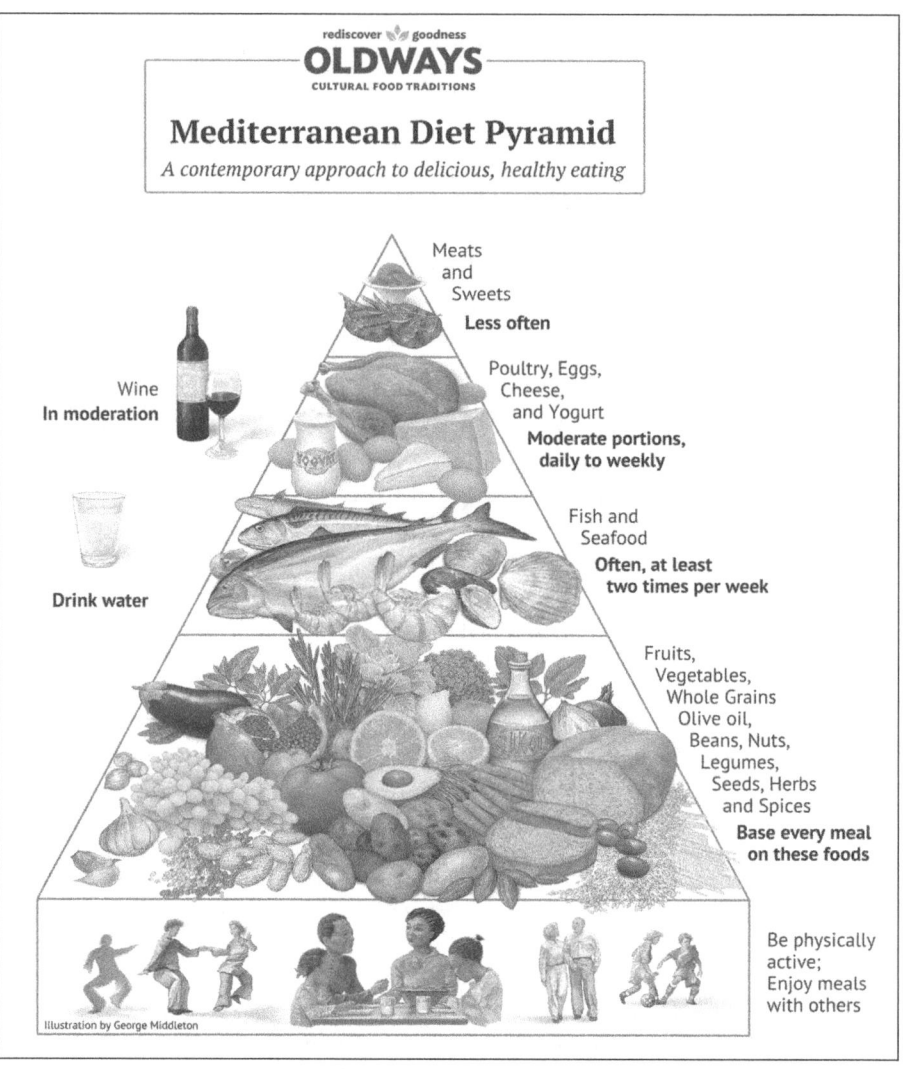

FIGURE 12-1:
The
Mediterranean
Diet Pyramid.

Treating prediabetes and other illnesses

For prediabetes and glucose regulation, a substantial and consistent body of evidence shows that adopting a Mediterranean-style eating pattern improves blood glucose control and reduces the risk of progression to Type 2 diabetes. Trials and long-term studies have found that Mediterranean-pattern diets are associated with lower rates of Type 2 diabetes, modest reductions in fasting glucose and HbA1C, and improvements in markers of insulin sensitivity compared with typical Western diets or low-fat diets. Those benefits are seen even when weight loss is modest or absent, because the pattern emphasizes high-fiber whole grains, legumes, vegetables and fruit, and healthy fats (including extra-virgin olive oil and nuts) that together produce steadier post-meal blood glucose responses. For people with established prediabetes, following this way of eating often reduces the likelihood of progressing to diabetes and can be a practical, sustainable component of an overall prevention plan.

Beyond glucose control, the Mediterranean diet delivers broad health benefits that lower the risk of many common chronic illnesses. Strong evidence links it to reduced rates of cardiovascular disease (fewer heart attacks, strokes and cardiovascular deaths), lower all-cause mortality, and improved control of blood pressure and blood lipids. It can be a fundamental part of successfully managing cholesterol. You can find more information in *Managing Cholesterol For Dummies* (Wiley 2025). Observational studies and randomized trials also suggest protection against cognitive decline and dementia, better outcomes for metabolic-syndrome features, and lower levels of chronic inflammation, factors that influence a wide range of conditions. Some studies show associations with reduced risk for certain cancers and improvements in overall quality of life and functional health in older adults. Importantly, these benefits arise from a dietary pattern that is flexible, palatable and culturally adaptable, which helps people sustain the changes needed for long-term health gains rather than short-term fixes.

Recognizing the environmental benefits of the Mediterranean diet

The Mediterranean diet is recognized as an environmentally sustainable way of eating because it emphasizes plant-based foods, such as vegetables, fruits, legumes, nuts, and whole grains, while limiting the intake of red meat and processed foods. Research shows that greater adherence to the Mediterranean diet is linked to reduced greenhouse gas emissions, lower land and water use, and less energy consumption compared to diets higher in animal products. By shifting away from diets high in red meat toward the Mediterranean pattern, there is potential to stabilize climate impact, conserve wildlife, and reduce conversion of land for agriculture. Adopting a Mediterranean-style diet not only benefits personal and public health but also contributes to global efforts to protect biodiversity and promote sustainability.

Olive trees act as a significant carbon sink, meaning they absorb and store more carbon dioxide from the atmosphere than is released during the production of olive oil, making olive groves a contributor to reducing greenhouse gas emissions overall. They are also very drought-resistant and require less water than many other oil crops, such as soybeans or corn, enabling olive cultivation to have a lower water footprint even in times of scarcity. With good agricultural practices, olive oil production can also support soil conservation, promote biodiversity, and play a role in regenerative agriculture.

Making the diet affordable

Concerns about the cost of eating healthily can be a barrier for many people considering a change in diet and lifestyle, but research suggests that the Mediterranean diet need not be more expensive than a typical Western diet. It may even save money. A 2013 study in the United States involving sixty-three participants found that those who adopted a plant-based Mediterranean-style eating pattern, with an emphasis on cooking with extra virgin olive oil, reduced their usual grocery spend by around thirty US dollars each week. Participants not only spent less overall but also reduced purchases of less healthy products such as carbonated soft drinks, while achieving benefits such as weight loss.

Similar findings emerged from a 2017 randomized controlled trial in Australia, which included a detailed cost analysis of twenty participants. In this study, following a Mediterranean diet was actually more affordable than the participants' baseline eating patterns, with an average reduction in grocery costs of around 26 Australian dollars per week. A study from the University of South Australia published in 2023 found that a family of four could save approximately 28 Australian dollars each week by following a Mediterranean-style diet instead of a Western diet high in processed foods, sodium, and saturated fats. In the UK context, research has shown that high adherence to a Mediterranean diet was associated with a very small increase in daily food costs, roughly £0.20 per day (about 5.4 percent), or £1.40 per week. Importantly, much of that modest extra spending went toward higher quality components such as vegetables, fruits, and fish, while less was spent on more expensive, and less healthy items such as processed meats and sweets. These findings challenge the perception that a Mediterranean-style diet is a "luxury" option; in practice, basing meals around seasonal vegetables, legumes, whole grains, and other plant-based staples, supplemented with modest amounts of fish, dairy, and poultry, can be both health-promoting and budget-friendly.

Shining a light on extra virgin olive oil

Extra virgin olive oil is at the very heart of the Mediterranean diet, not just as a cooking fat but as a daily staple that underpins its flavor, character, and many of its health benefits. In traditional Mediterranean regions, it's common for each person to consume around three to five tablespoons per day, used for cooking, drizzling over vegetables and salads, and dipping bread. High-quality extra virgin olive oil is one of the more expensive ingredients in this dietary pattern, reflecting the care, time, and expertise needed to produce it and to preserve the most important beneficial anti-inflammatory and antioxidant compounds including polyphenols. When it is the main source of fat in the diet and is combined with abundant vegetables, legumes, and whole grains, it becomes a cost-effective choice within an overall affordable way of eating. A single bottle can last for many meals, elevating simple, inexpensive dishes with richness, depth of flavor, and powerful antioxidants. This combination of culinary enjoyment and health protection makes extra virgin olive oil a key ingredient worth prioritizing.

Discovering How the Mediterranean Diet Works

The Mediterranean diet has been shown to be beneficial for prediabetes and improve glucose regulation by reducing high peaks in sugar absorption and improving the insulin response through:

>> **Having a low glycemic index (GI) and load.** Many core foods such as legumes, whole grains, and most whole fruits release sugar slowly, while healthy fats and proteins further lower the meal's glycemic load, preventing sharp blood glucose spikes. This facet is explored in more detail in the following section.

>> **Improving insulin sensitivity.** The healthy monounsaturated and polyunsaturated fats common in the diet, for example from olive oil, nuts, and oily fish help cells respond better to insulin, reduce harmful fat in the liver and muscles, and protect insulin-producing cells.

>> **Reducing insulin resistance.** Regular consumption of Mediterranean foods is linked to lower fasting insulin helping the body regulate glucose more effectively, especially when more insulin is needed following a meal.

>> **Decreasing oxidative stress and inflammation.** Antioxidants and anti-inflammatory compounds from extra virgin olive oil, vegetables (especially a variety of colored plants), fruits, herbs, spices nuts and seeds, reduce free radical damage and inflammation that impair insulin action.

>> **Supporting a healthy gut microbiome.** Fiber and polyphenol rich foods promote beneficial gut bacteria that produce short-chain fatty acids, improving gut health, reducing inflammation, and supporting insulin sensitivity.

>> **Encouraging healthy body weight and fat distribution.** High satiety (the feeling of fullness after a meal) from fiber, protein, and healthy fats supports achieving and maintaining a healthy weight while reducing visceral fat that worsens insulin resistance.

>> **Enhancing food synergy and nutrient combinations.** Combining healthy fats (such as extra virgin olive oil) with carbohydrates slows sugar absorption and lowers post-meal glucose rises, while improving nutrient absorption from vegetables.

>> **Improving lipid profile and reducing ectopic fat.** The diet lowers triglycerides and raises HDL cholesterol, reducing fat deposits in the liver and muscles, which improves insulin sensitivity.

>> **Supporting hormonal regulation.** Improves post-meal hormone responses such as GLP-1, which help regulate appetite, insulin release, and blood sugar.

>> **Changing gene expression through epigenetic effects.** Bioactive compounds, especially polyphenols from extra virgin olive oil, nuts, grapes, and berries, can influence gene activity, turning on genes that improve insulin signaling and turning off those linked to inflammation and oxidative stress.

REMEMBER

The regulation of blood glucose is much more complex than simply modifying amount of carbohydrates. The fats and proteins in foods as well as the micronutrients and other bioactive compounds play a major part in glucose regulation.

Carbohydrates and GI Index

Carbohydrates are the main source of sugar in our diet and are an important part of our diet, but in the Mediterranean diet they come mainly from minimally processed, high-fiber sources such as whole grains, legumes, vegetables, and fruits. These foods provide complex carbohydrates that are digested more slowly than refined, processed starches and sugars, leading to a steadier release of glucose into the bloodstream. The fiber in unprocessed wholegrain carbohydrates plays a central role here, especially the soluble, "viscous" type found in oats, beans, lentils, and some fruits, which forms a gel in the gut that slows the absorption of sugar. This fiber not only helps keep blood glucose levels more stable but also supports a healthy gut microbiome and promotes satiety, which can help with weight control. Wholegrain choices such as brown rice instead of white rice, whole meal or multigrain bread instead of white bread, steel-cut or rolled oats instead of instant oats, whole wheat pasta instead of regular pasta, and whole barley or quinoa instead of their refined, polished, or pearled versions provide more fiber, nutrients, and cause a slower, steadier rise in blood sugar.

TIP

Traditional grains used in minimally processed breads such as barley, rye, and spelt are a better choice than modern industrial wheat varieties in standard bread. They have higher fiber levels and intact grain components (bran, germ, and endosperm) that are preserved rather than removed through processing, resulting in a slower rise in blood glucose and also making them easier to digest for some people.

A useful way to understand the effects of carbohydrate foods on blood glucose is through the concepts of the glycemic index (GI) and glycemic load (GL). The glycemic index measures how quickly a food raises blood glucose compared with pure glucose, with high-GI foods causing a rapid spike and low-GI foods producing a slower, more gradual rise. The glycemic load takes this a step further by also considering how much carbohydrate a typical serving of food contains. For example, watermelon has a relatively high GI but a low GL because it contains little carbohydrate per serving. In the Mediterranean diet, many carbohydrate foods naturally have a low GI, and meals often combine carbohydrates with healthy fats and proteins, such as drizzling extra virgin olive oil on vegetables or bread which further lowers the overall glycemic load of the meal. This combination helps prevent the sharp blood sugar surges that can worsen insulin resistance and is one reason why the diet is so effective for managing prediabetes.

Plant proteins

Protein in the Mediterranean diet comes from a variety of sources, with a strong emphasis on plant-based proteins such as beans, lentils, chickpeas, peas, and nuts, alongside moderate amounts of fish, seafood, poultry, eggs, and smaller portions of dairy. These protein-rich foods help regulate blood sugar in several ways. They slow digestion and the absorption of carbohydrates, reducing the speed at which glucose enters the bloodstream after a meal. This helps avoid sudden spikes in blood glucose. Proteins also stimulate the release of hormones that promote satiety, making it easier to manage calorie intake and portion sizes and maintain a healthy weight, a key factor in improving insulin sensitivity.

Plant-based proteins have other benefits for glucose regulation because they are often packaged with fiber, and bioactive compounds such as polyphenols that reduce inflammation and oxidative stress. For example, lentils and chickpeas provide both protein and slow-digesting carbohydrates, leading to a gentler impact on blood glucose than refined grains or sugars. Nuts not only contribute protein but also supply healthy fats and bioactive compounds that further improve insulin function. In the Mediterranean diet, replacing some animal protein, especially red and processed meat with these plant-based sources can reduce saturated fat intake, improve lipid profiles, and lower the chronic inflammation that drives insulin resistance.

Fats

The Mediterranean diet is rich in healthy fats, mainly from plant-based sources such as extra-virgin olive oil, nuts, and seeds, as well as omega-3 fats from oily fish. These fats play a crucial role in improving glucose regulation and managing prediabetes. Monounsaturated fats (MUFA) and polyunsaturated fats (PUFA) help improve the way insulin works in the body and reduce the build-up of fat in the liver and muscles that can make the body less responsive to insulin.

These healthy foods also contain bioactive compounds such as polyphenols that reduce inflammation and oxidative stress — two key factors that interfere with insulin function. Consuming these fats improve cholesterol profiles by lowering triglycerides and raising HDL ("good") cholesterol, and the polyphenols reduce the oxidation of cholesterol which makes it particularly harmful for blood vessels. Including healthy fats with carbohydrate-rich meals slows digestion and sugar absorption, helping to prevent sharp rises in blood glucose after eating.

Polyphenols and bioactive compounds

Bioactive compounds are natural substances found in plant foods that are produced by the plant to protect itself from environmental stresses such as infections and oxidation — a chemical process where molecules lose electrons, involving damage from harmful reactive oxygen species that can damage plant cells and tissues, a process that is enhanced by heat and light. These protective antioxidants have beneficial effects on the body beyond basic nutrition. One important group of bioactive compounds in the Mediterranean diet are called polyphenols and are abundant in extra-virgin olive oil, fruits, vegetables, nuts, legumes, and berries. The Mediterranean diet is especially rich in these polyphenols, making it one of the most powerful dietary patterns for delivering these health-promoting compounds.

Polyphenols help improve blood sugar regulation in several ways. They enhance insulin sensitivity, meaning they help the body's cells respond better to insulin and use glucose more effectively. Polyphenols also reduce inflammation and oxidative stress, two major factors that can damage insulin function and contribute to prediabetes. They promote a healthy gut microbiome by encouraging beneficial bacteria that support metabolism and reduce harmful inflammation. Emerging research suggests polyphenols can even influence gene expression, turning on genes that improve insulin action and turning off those linked to inflammation and metabolic problems.

TIP

Because polyphenols are antioxidant compounds produced by plants and sometimes have a little pungency and bitterness taste as additional protection from being overeaten, foods from plants that have been grown under some degree of natural environmental stress are often richer in polyphenols. An example of this is the high level of polyphenols often seen in pleasantly bitter and pungent, well produced extra virgin olive oils which have been harvested early, been stored protected from heat, light and oxygen which degrade the antioxidant polyphenols, and are enjoyed as fresh as possible.

Other diets for prediabetes

You may come across other diets recommended for prediabetes, and some have evidence that they work through reducing carbohydrate and blood glucose load and improving insulin sensitivity, with more efficient regulation of blood glucose.

>> **DASH Diet (Dietary Approaches to Stop Hypertension).** Focuses on fruits, vegetables, whole grains, low-fat dairy, lean proteins, and limited sodium and added sugars. Originally designed for blood pressure control, it also helps improve insulin resistance and metabolic health.

It compares quite well with the Mediterranean diet, which is a naturally low salt diet with flavor gained from herbs and spices. Low-fat dairy is advised, however there is evidence that full fat dairy products especially the yogurt and unprocessed, authentic cheeses in the Mediterranean diet may actually reduce the risk of diabetes with no increase in cardiovascular diseases despite the saturated fat content.

>> **Low Glycemic Index (GI) diet.** Prioritizes foods that cause slower, steadier rises in blood glucose, such as whole grains, legumes, non-starchy vegetables, and most fruits. This helps avoid blood glucose spikes. The Mediterranean diet is by definition a low GI diet but with many additional benefits from its other key elements.

>> **Plant-based or vegetarian diets.** Emphasize plant foods with minimal animal products, increasing fiber and antioxidants intake while reducing saturated fat, supporting improved insulin sensitivity. The Mediterranean diet is plant predominant though does allow for the inclusion of meat and dairy products in moderation.

>> **Weight-loss focused diets.** Any calorie-controlled eating plan that promotes gradual weight loss, such as balanced low-calorie diets or structured programs, helps reduce insulin resistance and improve glucose control. However, unlike the Mediterranean diet, there is often no focus on improving health and well-being in parameters other than weight.

Low carbohydrate and low–calorie diets such as the paleo, Atkins and keto diets are promoted for weight loss, and with carbohydrate restriction glucose levels and HbA1c can fall.

WARNING

However, these types of diets have several problems. Advocating a reduction in a whole macronutrient group such as carbohydrates can result in the omission of healthy foods that belong to this group. Unprocessed vegetables and fruits are almost exclusively carbohydrates and, while they may vary in their glycemic index, they are fundamental to a good diet, with vitamins, minerals, fiber and bioactive compounds all contributing to health. Some carbohydrate restricting diets advise the replacement of carbs with meat or unhealthy fats, and whilst it's possible to reduce weight and HbA1c on such a regime, it is likely to increase levels of harmful cholesterol, oxidative stress and inflammation which may increase the risk of cardiovascular and other diseases. A dietary pattern needs to be enjoyable and sustainable in the long term, with research showing that people find low carbohydrate diets difficult to maintain in the long term. Finally, a diet which moves away from a plant predominant diet has a significantly higher impact on the environment.

It is better to be overweight and on a Mediterranean diet than to be following a nutritionally poor-quality dietary regime even if you lose weight with it.

Some expert-led programs for prediabetes may recommend a low carbohydrate diet, but when food groups are described, they actually do allow, and often encourage, the consumption of some low GI carbohydrates, especially vegetables and fruits with high fiber content. This factor can cause confusion because the term "low carbohydrate" diet can be misconstrued as being a paleo, keto, or Atkins style of diet, where carbohydrates are much more significantly reduced. There clearly is a difference between a carrot and a high sugar soda though both are "carbohydrates." Only one should be excluded from a healthy diet. The Mediterranean diet is not particularly low in carbs but the predominantly carbohydrate foods provide excellent nutrition and the whole diet ensures excellent glucose regulation.

Chapter **13**

Making the Mediterranean Diet Work for You

A t the time of writing this book, *U.S. News & World Report* has named the Mediterranean diet the number one diet in the world for its longstanding history, easiness to implement, and flexibility. The Mediterranean diet is not actually a simple diet, but rather a lifestyle, and the word "diet" itself derives from the Greek word *diaita,* which means way of life. We prefer this definition.

By choosing to adapt a Mediterranean lifestyle and implement it in your own way of living, you are selecting the optimal plan for achieving your health goals and preventing prediabetes from escalating. It is a lifestyle that, when followed, enables people to thrive and enjoy life much longer than others. Best of all, with enjoyable daily activities and delicious meals and recipes to choose from, the Mediterranean lifestyle enables you to enjoy yourself while following it.

A healthy diet is definitely one that sustainably supports people to achieve and maintain a healthy weight, but it must also deliver reduced risks of many chronic diseases including prevention or reversal of prediabetes. The advice in this book and *Diabetes For Dummies* (Wiley) can help and support everyone to adopt the healthiest of lifestyles to add quality years to life.

In this chapter, we share tips on how to incorporate the Mediterranean lifestyle into your life to enjoy both pleasure and good health.

The Lifestyle behind the Mediterranean Diet

Have you ever thought about how many toasts begin with "to health"? *L'chaim* in Hebrew, *Santè* in French, *Salud* in Spanish, *alla salute* in Italian, and so forth. Before Egyptians eat, they say "*bilhanna wi shefa*" which means "with pleasure and health." Chef Amy signs her books with that salutation, because it has become the mantra of her work, to ensure both. Luckily, the Mediterranean diet enables both.

First of all, if a diet or lifestyle is pleasurable, it's much more sustainable. Diets that cause you to completely abolish major food groups, sugar, or a favorite treat completely are probably ones that you won't be able to stick with. The same concept goes for physical activity. Lifestyle plans that require you to buy expensive equipment, spend hours in the gym, and do boring repetitive movements probably won't hold your attention for long. You can walk, swim, garden, bicycle, and even take the stairs for exercise instead.

The Mediterranean lifestyle is based on culture, principles, values, and foods that have enabled people to feel their best for thousands of years. It includes a deep respect for hospitality, pride in doing things yourself, a zeal for cooking for others, and a need for daily physical exercise. By adopting these beliefs as your own, you reap mental, physical, and spiritual benefits while healing yourself in the process.

Appreciating the Mediterranean Approach to Life

The Mediterranean lifestyle doesn't start with food. It starts with humans and mother nature, and their symbiotic relationship. While sociology and history are often left out of Mediterranean diet discussions, understanding a bit of their role in developing the millennia old, yet still highly effective lifestyle plan is imperative. The Mediterranean diet wasn't something that was invented in a laboratory or a classroom, it evolved over thousands of years to extract the best out of life.

Nowadays you can find glowing examples of the Mediterranean lifestyle in full effect everywhere from North Africa to Southern Europe to the Middle East. In this chapter, we introduce the common lifestyle denominators you can adapt to your own lifestyle with success no matter where you live. *Mediterranean Lifestyle For Dummies* by Amy Riolo (Wiley) can help you really explore the possibilities of this healthy diet and lifestyle.

Viewing food as a powerful ally

When thinking of food in the context of the Mediterranean lifestyle, remembering in the Mediterranean region that food is seen as an ally, not as an enemy to be avoided, is important. How many times have you personally heard the words "I'm on a diet, I can't even think about food!" That's because in modern societies we have so much excess food and calories at our disposal that we need to make significant efforts to eat less, and eat better, more wholesome foods when we want to take care of our health.

Thousands of years ago in the Mediterranean region, however, food wasn't so plentiful. The only options (thankfully) that people had were seasonal produce and grains, aged/fermented items such as cheese and vegetables that were preserved to last in the colder months, shelf stable nuts/seeds, beans and legumes, and yogurt or dairy as part of a daily diet. Fresh fish supplemented the diet as did the occasional portions of meat when an animal was slaughtered (this was not a daily occasion). Extra virgin olive oil, vinegar, and citrus juice dressed pretty much everything.

In those days no one had to worry about giving up processed and junk foods because they didn't exist yet. Heavy taxes were imposed on sugar and wheat as well as milling, so those items were historically hard to come by for everyone except the elite. Pharmaceuticals and medicines consisted of mixes made of herbs, flowers, resins, and spices. As a result, people associated foods with their health properties for millennia.

To this day, if you speak the local languages of different Mediterranean countries that you travel in, you will likely overhear someone recommending EVOO (extra virgin olive oil) and wild thyme to someone with a cough or chest congestion, anise seed tea to someone with a sore throat, ginger to someone with an upset stomach, and so on. Different countries, communities, and even households have their own traditional remedies, but one factor is common; food is seen and used as an ally.

People in the Mediterranean region familiarize themselves with the type of nutrients that they need (especially as they are going through various life cycles) and attempt to incorporate them into their diet. They uphold a strong preference for homemade food, even if they can afford to dine out wherever they'd like. For this reason, the Mediterranean diet is made up of a variety of the essential nutrients that those who follow a standard American diet or other western diets are likely to miss out on.

One of those nutrients is *dietary fiber,* which is a key component of the Mediterranean diet. Throughout history this source of fiber came along with carbohydrates and other key nutrients from unrefined grains, legumes (beans and peas), fresh fruits, and vegetables. Even though we don't have to pay heavy taxes on wheat or milling today, it's still a healthier option to choose less processed whole grains as a part of our daily diet.

One benefit of dietary fiber is simply making you feel full sooner and for a longer period between meals. A satisfied appetite often leads to consuming fewer calories, and avoiding unhealthy culinary temptations, which can lead to weight loss. Notice the different types of whole grains used in the recipes in Chapter 15. Whenever centenarians are interviewed in Italy — they are always asked what they eat and what they ate throughout their life. In every interview we see, they always mention whole grains and legumes as being main staples in their diets.

Legumes — beans, chickpeas, peas, and lentils — are a key source of low-fat protein in a Mediterranean diet and are a rich source of soluble fiber. They are the "Mediterranean" food that is most lacking from American diets. This omission is an easy fix, however, because legumes are readily available around the world, inexpensive, and easy to prepare a variety of ways. Soluble fiber helps reduce cholesterol, especially LDL (bad) cholesterol, a key risk factor for heart disease. Whole grain consumption is associated with lower blood pressure, even in relatively small amounts. High blood pressure along with diabetes is a double whammy for your kidneys, as well as a risk factor for heart disease and stroke. Aim to eat a serving of legumes each day.

If the idea of consistently eating beans and grains sounds bland to you, you're in for a surprise. You can transform these humble ingredients into soups, stews, patties, sandwiches, pasta, and rice dishes, and much more. Think of them instead as a blank culinary canvas with which you can paint a beautiful Mediterranean dish with flavor enhancers such as vinegars, capers, rosemary, mushrooms, citrus, mint, garlic, honey, fennel, peppers, cumin, paprika, onions, saffron, thyme, tomatoes, sage, bay leaf, oregano, nuts, dill, yogurt — to name just a few.

Best of all, each of these flavor boosting items contains powerful nutritional benefits. Discovering to harness their power adds another layer of taste and nutrients.

HARNESSING THE POWER OF CULINARY MEDICINE FOR PREDIABETES

Culinary medicine is a modern term used to describe the intersection of the culinary arts and nutrition. The truth of the matter is that human beings have been eating healing foods in specific combinations to promote health and longevity for thousands of years. What we now call culinary medicine was simple a way of life before the processed food and drug industry was born. Cooks knew which ingredients to use to boost health, and because they only had fresh, seasonal ingredients to choose from, they naturally started off with an advantage. If we fast forward to modern times, we can use science to back up the claims of the health benefits of eating plant-based foods.

Did you know that thousands of bioactive compounds are found in fruits and vegetables that we often enjoy including polyphenols, carotenoids, and glucosinolates? The antioxidant and anti-inflammatory effects of these "good for you" chemicals may have a significant effect on reversing prediabetes and the risk of Type 2 diabetes as well as many other chronic illnesses. The Mediterranean diet is naturally rich in bioactive compounds and has been shown to reduce the markers of chronic inflammation which is at the roots of all illness.

In Table 13-1 created by Dr Simon Poole, we can see the different types of polyphenols available in foods and the benefits that they offer. Nowadays culinary schools are starting to teach culinary medicine to chefs so that they can be certified in a healing style of cuisine. Chef Amy has been a longtime proponent of this philosophy and now uses Dr. Poole's table as a point of reference when she creates recipes for her health-centered cookbooks and in the recipes in Chapter 15.

TABLE 13-1　**C-1 Polyphenols in Foods and Possible Bioactivity**

Polyphenol Class	Polyphenol Type	Example	Food Sources	Potential Health Benefits
Flavonoids	Flavonols	Quercetin	Onions, apples, berries, broccoli, green tea, capers, citrus fruits	Antioxidant, anti-inflammatory, cardiovascular health, allergy relief
Flavonoids	Flavonols	Kaempferol	Kale, spinach, broccoli, green tea, strawberries, fennel	Antioxidant, anti-inflammatory, cardiovascular health, anticancer properties

(continued)

TABLE 13-1 *(continued)*

Polyphenol Class	Polyphenol Type	Example	Food Sources	Potential Health Benefits
Flavonoids	Flavonols	Myricetin	Berries, grapes, red wine, pomegranate, walnuts, red onions	Antioxidant, anti-inflammatory, brain health, anticancer properties
Flavonoids	Flavanols (Catechins)	Epicatechin	Green tea, cocoa, red wine, apples, berries, cherries, pears	Antioxidant, cardio-vascular health, blood sugar regulation
Flavonoids	Flavanols (Catechins)	Epigallocatechin gallate (EGCG)	Green tea, matcha, apples, berries, cocoa, dark chocolate	Antioxidant, metabolic health, brain health, weight management
Flavonoids	Flavanones	Hesperetin	Citrus fruits (oranges, lemons, grapefruits), tomatoes, parsley	Antioxidant, cardio-vascular health, anti-inflammatory
Flavonoids	Flavanones	Naringenin	Grapefruit, tomatoes, oranges, lemons, grapefruit juice, hops	Antioxidant, cardio-vascular health, metabolic health
Flavonoids	Flavones	Luteolin	Parsley, celery, chamomile tea, thyme, sage, peppermint	Antioxidant, anti-inflammatory, brain health, anticancer properties
Flavonoids	Flavones	Apigenin	Parsley, celery, chamomile tea, artichokes, basil, celery seed	Antioxidant, anti-inflammatory, brain health, anticancer properties
Flavonoids	Anthocyanins	Cyanidin	Blueberries, blackberries, cherries, grapes, cranberries, eggplant	Antioxidant, cardio-vascular health, brain health, anti-aging
Flavonoids	Anthocyanins	Delphinidin	Blueberries, cranberries, raspberries, blackcurrants, red radishes	Antioxidant, cardiovascular health, brain health, anti-inflammatory
Phenolic acids	Hydroxybenzoic acids	Gallic acid	Coffee, tea, blueberries, blackberries, strawberries, red wine	Antioxidant, anti-inflammatory, cardiovascular health, anticancer properties
Phenolic acids	Hydroxybenzoic acids	Protocatechuic acid	Green tea, apples, pears, cinnamon, cocoa, cherry, vanilla	Antioxidant, anti-inflammatory, metabolic health, brain health

Polyphenol Class	Polyphenol Type	Example	Food Sources	Potential Health Benefits
Phenolic acids	Hydroxycinnamic acids	Caffeic acid	Coffee, whole grains, apples, pears, artichokes, lettuce, parsnips	Antioxidant, anti-inflammatory, cardio-vascular health, anticancer properties
Stilbenes	Resveratrol	Resveratrol	Red grapes, red wine, peanuts, mulberries, dark chocolate, pistachios	Antioxidant, anti-inflammatory, cardio-vascular health, brain health
Other	Secoiridoides	Oleuropein, oleocanthal, Tyrosols	Extra virgin olive oil	Anti-inflammatory, cardiovascular health including oxidation of LDL cholesterol, anti-oxidant properties
Other	Lignans	Secoisolarici-resinol	Flaxseeds, sesame seeds, whole grains, berries, cruciferous vegetables	Antioxidant, hormonal balance, cardiovascular health, anticancer properties
Other	Lignans	Enterolactone	Flaxseeds, sesame seeds, whole grains, berries, cruciferous vegetables	Hormonal balance, anticancer properties, cardiovascular health

Fresh fruits and vegetables are so integral to the Mediterranean lifestyle that meals are actually planned around them. For example, many western and modern chefs and home cooks plan meals around meat, poultry, or fish. The (non-plant based) source of protein is usually the star of the meal. Vegetables and fruits are usually an afterthought. You can still create healthful meals this way, but it is much more difficult. Vegetable portions are usually smaller to compliment large pieces of meat — and fresh fruit gets forgotten about altogether.

In traditional Mediterranean meals — however, vegetables and fruit are considered first. Even in major cities, people everywhere from Marseille to Marrakesh, Athens, Rome, and Cairo can purchase fresh produce on the street and in all markets. It's easy to tell which ones are in season (that's mostly all they have) and consumers know that those ingredients are good for them. They may pick up some artichokes, fennel, persimmons, and citrus, for example. They then think of what they want to make with the artichokes — pasta, soup, stew, tajine, and so forth. The fennel and citrus can get turned into a beautiful salad, and the persimmons served after the meal for dessert (on a special occasion a more elaborate dessert would follow). Meat, fish, or poultry may get added in small amounts to the artichoke stew or tajine, but it isn't be the main event. That way, a person gets a minimum of four of the recommended 9-12 servings of fresh fruit and vegetables in one meal instead of one or two.

If you're serious about following the Mediterranean lifestyle, challenge yourself to incorporate as many fresh vegetables as possible with some fruit as a snack or dessert replacement. Leafy greens are especially important for those looking to reverse prediabetes or diabetes because they contain vitamins and minerals including magnesium, and other nutrients that help to balance blood sugar and keep you full.

Choose colorful vegetables to add an assortment of vitamins nutrients and bioactive compounds including polyphenols to the mix. Fresh fruit is the dessert of choice, and the fruits and vegetables should be enjoyed without added sugar, fat, or salt (sodium). The dietary fiber from this fruit and vegetable part of the Mediterranean diet, as well as from legumes and grains, can benefit your health in another very important way — blood glucose control, which is essential for those with prediabetes.

Living Mediterranean Style from Anywhere

In 2010, UNESCO recognized the Mediterranean diet to be an "Intangible Cultural Heritage of Humanity" and characterized it as "a set of skills, knowledge, practices, and traditions ranging from the landscape to the table, including the crops, harvesting, fishing, conservation, processing, preparation, and, particularly, consumption of food."

Living Mediterranean style is easy if you are in that part of the world. The lifestyle and local cultures dictate a health boosting and community centric pace that enables one to live better almost "accidentally." But what about following these healthful behaviors in Boston, Chicago, London, or another major city where the sun isn't always shining and people don't take two-hour lunch breaks followed by a siesta?

The short answer is simple, decide that this lifestyle can improve your health no matter where you live and vow to practice as many of its principles as possible. In the beginning you may feel like a fish out of water, and it may be hard to stick to your guns when no one around you is living this way. But you will experience payoff in the end, and your health and happiness may even inspire those around you to follow in your footsteps.

When Chef Amy first visited her relatives in Calabria, Italy, in the 1990s, she noticed that they were much healthier than their kin who had lived in the United States for decades. Even though the family members shared the same genes and traits, the Italian relatives were much healthier. It was at that time when she decided to identify, categorize, and preach the lifestyle habits that helped her Italian family to thrive. In the beginning it was just for her own American family's benefit. The Mediterranean diet wasn't known about in the United States back then. Little by little her passion turned into a career and a personal lifestyle. In her *Mediterranean Lifestyle For Dummies* book, she created the following "Getting a Mediterranean Lifestyle Checklist" — a four-and-a-half page guide that you can print out and keep at your desk or in your journal.

Read through the list and note which items you're already doing and then incorporate others which are easily within your reach. Make a conscious effort to add new items into your daily rituals each week. Many of the items on the list are free and easy to implement, but they offer numerous mental, spiritual, and physical benefits.

The Mediterranean diet has been long established, deeply rooted in ancient ways of living, and has continued to evolve, embracing new flavors of herbs and spices from the Far East along early trade routes as well as chocolate and tomatoes from the New World and coffee from Africa.

Getting a Mediterranean Lifestyle Checklist

- ❑ **Grow and use fresh herbs in your home or garden.** You can use a simple windowsill or a cart placed in front of a window to grow healthful herbs — you don't need a big yard.

- ❑ **Cook a meal for yourself and/or your family.** Take pleasure in making more of your meals at home and sharing them with others for the mental and physical payoff.

- ❑ **Decide who to eat with before deciding what to eat.** Eating communally is the backbone of the Mediterranean lifestyle — the more, the merrier!

- ❑ **Base each meal around produce.** Decide which fresh, local vegetables you love, and make them the base of your meals.

- ❑ **Buy organic groceries when possible.** Better-quality food leads to better health.

- ❑ **Eat with others as often as possible.** Look for creative ways to include other people in your mealtimes — even if it means going outside of familial bonds and using unconventional methods such as FaceTime and Skype to do so.

- ❑ **Engage in physical activity that you enjoy.** Doing what you love is as good for the psyche as physical exercise is for the body. Pick some activities you really enjoy, and you get total body benefits at the same time. If you add nature into the mix, you get three benefits at once!

- ❑ **Participate in a hobby or activity that you enjoy.** This activity adds meaning and pleasure in your life while contributing to your purpose and lowering stress.

- ❑ **Visit a farm.** Seeing where your food comes from helps you to be more in tune with what's seasonal and local. Often you can pick your own ingredients, which means more exercise and fresh air!

- ❑ **Attend a food festival.** Food festivals are a great way to celebrate local ingredients, discover new recipes, and support the community while spending time outdoors.

- ❑ **Try a new recipe.** This activity provides a sense of accomplishment while increasing your cooking skills and confidence.

- ❑ **Teach someone a new recipe.** Passing along knowledge is mentally satisfying and helps to boost relationships and camaraderie.

- ❑ **Bring or make a healthy lunch on workdays.** You enjoy nutritionally sound meals and save money.

- ❑ **Use good-quality extra virgin olive oil as your main cooking fat.** This healthful fat provides powerful antioxidants and omega-3 fatty acids, which work to coax additional nutrients out of healthful foods and have anti-inflammatory properties that help keep many diseases at bay.

- ❑ **Take a walk outdoors after a meal.** Walking after a meal improves digestion and increases your exposure to nature and the outdoors.

- ❑ **Spend time gardening or with potted plants.** A recent study revealed that gardening was linked to greater happiness along with eating out, biking, walking, and recreational activities.

- ❑ **Shop at a farmers' market when possible.** You can form relationships with local food providers, get access to the best foods available, and be part of your community.

- ❑ **Enjoy healthful foods as the base of each meal.** Make sure that your meals are based on healthful ingredients such as leafy greens, cruciferous vegetables, beans, legumes, whole grains, fish and seafood, and dairy, with good-quality meat eaten sparingly.

- ❑ **Use aromatics to flavor food.** Instead of adding more salt, butter, and cream to recipes to make your food taste better, opt for good-quality spices, handfuls of chopped fresh herbs, garlic, onions, and shallots to produce more taste without the calories and fat.

- ❑ **Create meat-free meals when possible.** Many Americans base their meals around meat. Swapping the meat out for fish, chicken, dairy, or plant-based protein (such as legumes and soy), even a few times a week, make a difference.

- ❑ **Choose fruit for dessert.** On regular days, instead of finishing a meal with a fat- and calorie-laden dessert, grab a piece of fresh fruit instead. You get a dose of sweetness along with vitamins and minerals. Save the super-sweet treats for special occasions or once a week.

- ❑ **Start or maintain a healthful eating ritual with friends or family.** If you can, start a tradition of eating at least one meal a day with friends, family, colleagues, or others who value the benefits of communal eating.

- ❑ **Add an additional serving of fish to your weekly diet.** Just one additional serving per week can reduce your risk of heart disease by 49 percent while providing healthful fats and brainpower-boosting nutrients.

- ❑ **Aim for five to 12 servings of fresh fruits and vegetables daily.** Eating lots of leafy green vegetables along with the "rainbow" of colors in produce every day is an easy way to fill up on fiber while ensuring that you're getting a wide range of nutrients.

- ❑ **Add leafy green vegetables to your lunch and dinner menus.** Artichokes, asparagus, avocado, broccoli, Brussels sprouts, cabbage, celery, chicory, collard greens, dandelion greens, kale, kiwi, lettuce, purslane, spinach, Swiss chard, and zucchini are examples of nutrient-dense produce. Be sure to add at least one of them to every meal.

- ❑ **Stock a pantry with healthful, Mediterranean options.** Turn to Chapter 14 for more information.

- ❑ **Create a week's worth of Mediterranean menus for each meal before making a shopping list.** Turn to Chapter 12 for more on this subject.

- ❑ **Bring healthful snacks, such as fruit and nuts, with you when you leave home.** This plan staves off hunger longer and ensures that you aren't satisfying your hunger with something unhealthy.

- ❑ **Listen to beautiful music whenever possible.** Music helps boost your mood, energy, and concentration. Grapes grow better and are more resistant to disease when classical music is played in vineyards, so imagine what it can do for your body!

- ❑ **Beautify your space with objects that are meaningful to you.** We all have our own definitions of beauty and what's meaningful to us. The more of those elements that you can add to your work and home space, the better.

- ❑ **Choose quality over quantity.** No matter the topic, quality always beats out quantity in the Mediterranean region. Older cultures appreciate things that last and are willing to have less variety in order to have something that will stand the test of time.

- ❏ **Talk with a close confidante.** Having someone to confide in is integral to mental health.

- ❏ **Get a minimum of 30 minutes of fresh air per day.** Mental health professionals claim that fresh air is more beneficial to our moods than antipsychotic drugs are.

- ❏ **Laugh as often as possible.** Lowering stress and increasing happiness is great for healing and preventing illness.

- ❏ **Make time for rest and relaxation.** Rest and relaxation are a daily, not a once-a-year, practice in the Mediterranean region.

- ❏ **Look on the bright side of situations that are bothersome in your life.** Making the best out of whatever life deals you is an art form in the Mediterranean.

- ❏ **Spend time in nature, preferably by water and/or green trees.** The "green effect" and the "blue effect" of spending just 10 minutes a day looking at trees or water have emotional benefits.

- ❏ **Practice gratitude for blessings large and small as often as possible.** "If you say only one prayer, make it thank you" is a popular philosophy in the region, and this attitude helps attract more of the things we love.

- ❏ **Live your purpose in every way possible.** This mindset adds meaning to your days and make living worthwhile.

- ❏ **Eat your larger meal at lunchtime.** In the middle of the day, you still have time to burn off more calories, and it will help you to maintain a healthier weight and sleep better.

- ❏ **Take a 10- to 20-minute nap.** Naps help productivity, focus, weight management, stress reduction, and much more.

- ❏ **Aim for six to eight hours of sleep every night.** Getting enough sleep promotes better overall body functions, such as blood sugar management, hormonal functions, and brain performance.

- ❏ **Create a DIY project.** Having a project promotes a sense of accomplishment and purpose.

- ❏ **Participate in a cultural activity (for example, theater, opera, or a sporting event) with loved ones.** Socialization increases the level of oxytocin (known as the "love hormone").

- ❏ **Host guests for a meal, coffee, or tea.** Even a small gesture goes a long way toward promoting feelings of camaraderie and community.

- ❏ **Organize your day around your meals as much as possible.** This ensures eating the right foods at the right times while promoting a sense of security and safety.

- **Drink herbal teas in the evening before bed and throughout the day.** The nutritional benefits of herbs can help in achieving our various health goals and are healthful, caffeine-free rituals.

- **Eat one serving of beans or legumes per day.** Most Americans fall short in this category, but these foods are an important part of the Mediterranean diet.

- **Spend some time in the sun.** Getting more vitamin D helps immunity, while sun exposure increases serotonin (a mood stabilizer).

- **Contribute to charity or volunteer your time.** In addition to helping the community, volunteering helps to increase oxytocin.

- **Peruse philosophy books.** Philosophy helps us to understand ourselves, the world we live in, and how we relate to it.

- **Practice ethical and/or spiritual traditions that are symbolic to you.** These traditions add meaning, ritual, and routine to life, while offering support mechanisms during times of adversity.

- **Cook with as many local ingredients as possible.** Our bodies crave the nutrients found in produce that's in season in the regions we live in. In addition to saving money and supporting the environment, eating locally is better for your health.

- **Engage in community efforts as often as possible.** Strong community relationships provide psychological security and advantages.

- **Foster fabulous friendships.** Having a few trustworthy friends and confidents is important for mental well-being.

- **Strive for authenticity in your relationships.** Being genuine and sincere is the best way to foster healthy relationships.

Fitting the Mediterranean Diet into Your Life

Mediterranean diet lexicon

No matter where you spend time in the Mediterranean, certain attitudes, practices, and beliefs contribute to the healthfulness of the Mediterranean lifestyle at large. Table 13-2 is a lexicon created by Chef Amy based on her time living, working, and traveling through the Mediterranean region. These items are often left out of nutritional discussions which focus simply on what you should eat.

You can eat very healthful foods, and of course that's better than eating processed food. But if you eat those foods without these lifestyle elements, they won't have nearly the same mental, physical, or spiritual benefits as they do by adopting the beliefs below and practicing them.

Incorporate as many of these aspects into your life for best results while following a Mediterranean diet.

TABLE 13-2   ## The ABC's of the Mediterranean Lifestyle

Agriculture	Sustainable traditions yield better food.
Bread and **B**eauty	Bread is the backbone of the diet and culinary culture. Beauty is a concept valued by everyone in each area of daily life.
Community and **C**ulture	Acting, thinking, and eating for the benefit of the community and in a way that promotes cultural traditions.
D (the vitamin)	The sun provides a lot of vitamin D naturally.
Extra virgin olive oil	Extra virgin olive oil is the go-to cooking fat, flavor enhancer, and traditional medicinal.
Fresh air	Fresh air is prized for its health benefits.
Gardening	Most people in the Mediterranean enjoy gardening, whether on a balcony, on a rooftop, on a windowsill, or in a garden.
Home cooking	Home cooking is valued and prized for its important role in our overall health and in maintaining a culture's customs.
Inclusion	"The more the merrier" is usually the rule of thumb, and togetherness is preferred to being alone.
Joy	Joy is the ultimate daily goal and the reason for adopting as many pleasurable activities as possible.
Kin	Family matters most throughout the Mediterranean.
Laughter	Laughter is a natural remedy used to lift the spirits as often as possible.
Music	Music is an important part of every Mediterranean culture and enjoyed daily, not just on special occasions.
Nature	Nature is beloved, and people go the extra mile to preserve their communities' environments.
Outdoors	In the Mediterranean, people spend as much time outdoors or with a view of the outdoors as possible.
Purpose, **P**roduce, and **P**lants	A reason for living can be personal or collective, but knowing and acting on your purpose is essential for happiness to most people in the region. Fresh fruits and vegetables make up the bulk of the diet. Cultivate as many plants as possible — both for personal gratification and for the environment.

Quality	Quality is always chosen over quantity.
Rest and **R**elaxation	Rest and relaxation are important daily practices.
Sunlight	Sunlight leads to a sunny disposition and optimism. Seasonal affective disorder is not an issue in the Mediterranean region because people intentionally plan ways to incorporate more sun into their days, even in the winter months.
Traditions	Many people in the Mediterranean are working diligently to promote traditions from previous generations for the future as a means of preserving culture, identity, and more.
Unity	In the Mediterranean, a premium is placed on doing things together. This tradition has deep roots in maintaining peace between tribes and within communities. People work diligently to create common ground among those who have differing viewpoints instead of avoiding sensitive topics.
Value	Price is not the only way to measure the worth of an activity or object. Value in the Mediterranean region is assigned to things that enhance life, health, the environment, and the community, and people are willing to pay more money for those things.
Water	In addition to hydrotherapy, the healing effects of water and drinking enough from clean sources — often mineral springs — are promoted.
Xenia	*Xenia* is the Ancient Greek concept of hospitality, which is at the core of every Mediterranean culture. Locals strive to be good hosts in the way that other cultures may strive to win an award or get a promotion. The role of a host is taken very seriously, and to be a good host speaks to a person's character.
Young at heart	In an area that is home to many centenarians and highly functioning elderly people, keeping a youthful attitude is important. Letting go of concerns easily and fostering a childlike wonder for life are key factors.
Zeal	My Greek friends and I call this the "opa!" factor for the Greek exclamation that connotes a zest for life. A deep appreciation for life itself and a desire to live it to the fullest are commonplace in the region.

Ingredient swap outs for the Mediterranean diet

To truly enjoy the Mediterranean diet and lifestyle, you should plan your meals around ingredients and foods that hail from that region. With the wide range of flavor profiles and recipes that hail from the South of France through Italy, Greece, Lebanon, Turkey, Spain, Morocco, and Egypt (and that's just for starters), you won't get bored, and your palate will be more than pleased.

If you follow a traditional Mediterranean diet and steer clear of processed foods you won't need to make many swap outs. The recipes in this book keep you on the right track. We prefer you to start out with recipes which are already within the Mediterranean style, rather than trying to make those from the Standard

American Diet fit into the Mediterranean one, but there are times when you're getting started, traveling, or eating out, that swap outs can become useful. If that's the case, here are some substitutions to keep in mind:

Standard American Diet	Mediterranean Diet
Sour cream/Mayo	Plain Greek yogurt
Seed oils	Extra virgin olive oil
Butter	Extra virgin olive oil
Processed cereals	Whole grains
High fat red meat	Fish, seafood, chicken, turkey
Milk chocolate	Dark chocolate
Canned fruit and veg	Fresh fruits and veg
Salad dressings	EVOO/lemon juice/vinegar
Canned/boxed stocks	Homemade stocks or water
Soda/sweetened drinks/juices	Water
Snack bars/protein bars	Handful of unsalted almonds/three oz. piece Parmigiano-Reggiano cheese/½ cup plain Greek yogurt
Sugar	Raw honey
Crudites with dips	Crudites with homemade hummus
French fries	Herb and olive oil roasted potatoes
Table salt	Unrefined sea salt — fresh herbs and spices for flavor

These suggestions may not look like much, but if you currently eat a western diet or live in America and eat the foods on the left of the chart, incorporating the ones on the right in their place alone can make a big difference in your diet and blood glucose levels. Avoid as much processed food as possible. The hidden sugar and sweeteners in these foods is what causes many people to have a prediabetes diagnosis to begin with.

Greek yogurt can be used in baking as a replacement for sour cream and mayo. It can also be used to top potatoes, as a dip, and so on. Try adding fresh herbs and your favorite spices to make it even tastier.

We love extra virgin olive oil so much that we even wrote a book about it. See *Olive Oil For Dummies* (Wiley, 2025) to discover all the great ways that EVOO can improve your health, life, and recipes. You can bake with EVOO and cook with it. Chef Amy uses it in everything from traditional Mediterranean recipes to deep-frying, to making banana bread. Don't buy in to the old myths about not being able to heat extra virgin olive oil to high heats or that baking with it will change flavor. It will enhance it and make it healthier.

Making your own broth or stock instead of relying on those with high sodium contents is also a wonderful swap out. (See the Minestrone recipe in Chapter 15.) If Chef Amy doesn't have homemade stock on hand, she actually prefers to use water with additional fresh herbs and spices instead of boxed or canned stock for health reasons and flavor.

If you're not already doing so, vow to use extra virgin olive oil and lemon juice or vinegar — you can add some unsweetened Dijon mustard to the mix for texture if you like instead of prepared commercial salad dressings which are known to be full of fat, additives, and sweeteners. If those aren't satisfying enough for you, consider switching up your fresh salad ingredients to more tasty ones — such as those in the Nicoise Salad in Chapter 15. We'd rather you used the calories on high quality ingredients which help balance your blood sugar than unhealthful purchased dressings that will sabotage your meal plan.

By making these simple adjustments you are doing yourself a huge favor and taking major steps toward your health and better glucose control.

Chapter **14**

Incorporating the Mediterranean Lifestyle into Your Daily Routine

The Mediterranean lifestyle is a perfect example of a diet and life plan you can live happily with, not a diet you go on for a short period of time. The Mediterranean diet is a general pattern of eating which developed over millennia in the countries that surround the Mediterranean basin but can easily be implemented anywhere around the world (see Chapter 13). Following the Mediterranean lifestyle can lead to reduced inflammation, weight loss, reduce the risk of heart disease, increase longevity, reduce incidence and symptoms of Parkinson's and Alzheimer's diseases, prevent cancer and tumor growth, reduce the risk of death from heart disease and stroke and prevent and reverse hyperattention, ADHD, obesity, and most importantly for the readers of this book, diabetes.

In this chapter, you discover how the Mediterranean lifestyle can be incorporated into your daily life.

Planning to Start the 7-Day Routine

If eating and socializing with friends, getting pleasurable exercise and fresh air, taking pride in what you eat and cooking are already important parts of your life, then congratulations, when coupled with the right foods, you are already living Mediterranean-style. If they're not, then there's room for improvement. Coupled with a healthful and delicious diet you can enjoy these items and live Mediterranean style from anywhere.

In terms of diet, fresh, seasonal vegetables and fruits with extra-virgin olive oil being the main source of healthy fat. Unsalted nuts, minimally processed whole grains, milk, and yogurt are also base ingredients that should be enjoyed daily. Weekly consumption includes seafood, eggs, poultry, and lean meats. Red meat and sweets are limited to occasional consumption. If you pick any country in the Mediterranean — from Southern Europe to North Africa to the Middle East and look back to what people were eating on the average day 75 to 100 years ago — this what you will find. Pasta, whole grain bread, or other grains with vegetables and legumes enhanced with herbs and spices were the go-to meals of choice. On larger weekly meals (Friday in Muslim countries, Saturday in Jewish communities, and Sunday in Christian ones) people would eat larger meals, include seafood or meat if it was available, and often finish with a dessert. Daily sweet treats consisted of fresh or dried fruit.

The ingredients that people ate a century ago and for millennia prior may sound boring to modern diners, but if you think of how they came together to form some of our favorite foods, you can appreciate them more. Those same whole grains, vegetables, and legumes came together to form delectable, comforting dishes that have stood the test of time and place. Italian pasta e fagioli the Barley, Bean, and 5 Vegetable Minestrone and Whole Wheat Pasta with Creamy Lentil Sauce and Pecorino Cheese featured in Chapter 15 of this book are born out of that tradition. So is homemade hummus with whole wheat pita bread. Ubiquitous forms of bean and rice dishes beloved from Venice to Spain to Morocco and Egypt were born out of pantry staples and scores of them can keep you healthy and your palate satisfied.

Nuts and yogurt are great go-to snacks or breakfasts when paired with a piece of fresh fruit. A single serving of fish per week can greatly decrease your risk of heart disease, and eggs are a great source of protein. Keep in mind that one egg is a complete serving when it comes to eggs. Many American diners would have you think that three eggs is appropriate for breakfast — but it's actually the amount of eggs you should be eating over three days — not in one sitting. In the Mediterranean region — especially the Southern European countries such as Italy and Spain — eggs are turned into *frittata* and *tortas* and served at lunch or dinner instead of breakfast as a protein.

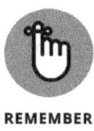

REMEMBER

The Mediterranean lifestyle doesn't require that you completely give up anything other than processed junk food. If you love steak or roasted meat, or a sugary dessert, enjoy a serving weekly to keep yourself on track and allow the simple pleasures.

Many sources tell you that people didn't eat meat historically in the Mediterranean because it was expensive. In many places in the Mediterranean meat was (and is still) much more expensive than it generally is in the United States. But that isn't the reason why people ate less of it. Daily meat or fish consumption was never "a thing" in the Mediterranean. The diet was truly based on vegetables, whole grains, dairy, and legumes. People would sacrifice an animal at holiday times or to honor special guests, and at that time it would be enjoyed. Not to be wasteful, they would consume the entire animal and preserve portions of it by curing or smoking it. Portions of that cured or smoked meat would be eaten throughout the year and added to soups and stews for flavor. But recognizing that no one wanted or thought about eating meat daily is important. In the west, that is a modern trend just like the obsession with consuming tremendous amounts of protein is.

TIP

Another common denominator among the people of the Mediterranean is a strong sense of faith. Personal differences and religious affiliations differed throughout the Mediterranean, but most people always had some sort of spiritual philosophy which superseded their own personal tastes that set the stage for their dietary choices. Nowadays, even in the Mediterranean, religious mandates aren't always followed as strictly as they were a century ago, and people often bend the rules. We like to suggest that regardless of your religious beliefs, when embarking upon the Mediterranean diet, that you accept it at a philosophical level. Whether you're a fan of Epicurus, Pythagoras, or Hippocrates, believe that taking care of your body is your divine duty, or simply want to "buy in" to a proven nutritional framework, become a "convert" to the ways of the Mediterranean will help you live longer and better.

The Mediterranean diet is deeply rooted in ancient ways of living, and has continued to evolve, embracing new flavors of herbs and spices from the Far East along early trade routes as well as chocolate and tomatoes from the New World and coffee from Africa. Even nowadays as Americans are attempting to embrace the diet, ingredients such as salmon and quinoa are making their way back to the Mediterranean to be incorporated in daily diets there. You don't need to limit your diet to what people were eating thousands of years ago. Thousands of years of culinary exchange have enhanced the "diet" to make it highly appealing today. In fact, if you were to serve traditional Mediterranean-style foods at a party, most people would just comment on how tasty they are, without even considering the health aspect.

To start on this lifestyle without moving to the Mediterranean region, here are some suggestions:

>> Decide *who* to eat with before deciding *what* to eat.

>> Make sure that most of your meals and snacks consist of fruits and vegetables, preferably unprocessed and whole.

>> If you eat bread or cereal, make sure that it's whole grain and artisanal. The same is true for rice and pasta. Many manufacturers now use special heirloom grains, which have less gluten and lower glycemic indexes.

>> Skip butter and use olive oil on everything instead.

>> Dress your salads with extra-virgin olive oil and lemon juice or good-quality vinegar only. Or use tahini (blended sesame seeds) as a dressing.

>> Eat a handful of raw unsalted almonds and a few good-quality olives prior to meals.

>> Add lots of fresh herbs, spices, and lemon juice to flavor your foods instead of extra salt and fat.

>> Grill or bake fish, poultry, and meat instead of frying or breading it.

>> Choose fish such as tuna, salmon, trout, mackerel, and herring. Check with www.SeafoodWatch.org to find out the most sustainable and safe seafood options prior to purchasing because the list changes often.

>> Try to eat a variety of flavors, textures, and colors in your food each day. When choosing produce, try to "eat the rainbow" as much as possible because different colored items contain different vitamins, minerals, and other nutrients as well as the all-important polyphenols. Enjoy spicy and bitter flavor contrasts especially from herbs and spices as this often denotes good levels of polyphenols.

Refer to *Mediterranean Lifestyle For Dummies* by Amy Riolo and *Diabetes Meal Planning and Nutrition* by Amy Riolo and Dr. Simon Poole (John Wiley & Sons, Inc.) for more information.

Seven-Day Mediterranean routine

This 7-day plan is based on a Monday–Sunday week where Monday–Friday are work days and Saturdays and Sundays are the weekend — but this model can be adapted to different work schedules as well as different calendars.

Every day take time to briefly look at the meal planning, food recommendations and recipes in this book and embrace the wonderful foods of the Mediterranean diet with plentiful colored vegetables, fruits, wholegrains, nuts, herbs, spices, and extra virgin olive oil.

In this exercise you are focusing specifically on one element each day to appreciate its power and potential to heal.

As you explore in detail a different aspect of the Mediterranean lifestyle during this 7-day plan, you will build healthy and enjoyable habits into each day. In the weeks, months and years that follow, you will find that you can incorporate these new habits into every week. If you find life seems to be getting in the way of any of the elements, it's perhaps time to remind yourself of their benefits by revisiting this 7-day plan.

Refer to the Mediterranean Lifestyle Checklist and reference in Chapter 13 for more specific ideas of ideas to work into your routine. The following is a very simple plan which can be tailored to your needs. It's based on techniques proven to promote optimal physical, mental, and emotional health, but you can personalize it to make sure that it works for your schedule and preferences.

Day One — Focus on conviviality

Throughout this book and all our work, we focus on the importance of socialization and spending time with others. The ancient Greek philosopher Epicurus was known for saying, "Look for someone to eat or drink with before looking for something to eat or drink." This statement underlines the importance of being in good company — giving it more importance than physical nourishment. Mediterranean cultures excel at conviviality (or friendliness) and it is one of the main reasons why the Mediterranean diet produced such great results.

In stark contrast, according to MDLinx, a news service for physicians "The newest epidemic in America (loneliness) now affects up to 47 percent of adults — double the number affected a few years ago. Preventing loneliness should be at the top of our list of priorities — right along with preventing diabetes and other illnesses. Today, focus on areas of your life which you could share with others. Whether it's eating together, going for a walk, having a coffee, playing a sport, or enjoying a shared activity, your health will improve by spending time with others. If you live or work alone, or are traveling, it is especially important to plan. Make plans with people, write them in your calendar and stick to them.

Follow the Schedule Base Template shown next.

Day Two — Focus on physical activity

Physical activity is another foundation of the Mediterranean diet pyramid. But if hours at the gym or using complicated equipment stresses you out, don't worry, you have many other ways to get in shape and burn calories. In fact, practicing types of physical activity that you enjoy helps you to stay on track and also improves your mood. Today, think about all the ways that you can get more physical activity. Read through Chapters 9 and 10 to familiarize yourself the different ways that you can achieve a healthy weight and live an active lifestyle.

Have you been longing to take dance lessons, try a new sport, go for more walks or on bike rides? Now's the time to start incorporating them into your schedule.

Follow the following Schedule Base Template.

Day Three — Focus on fresh air and nature

Getting fresh air and spending time outdoors can help to increase your overall outlook and physical health. Time outdoors boosts immunity, increases digestion, reduces your risk of illness, helps to balance hormones and promote better sleep and improves your mood. And that's just a few of the benefits. Aim for 30 minutes outdoors today, but if you can do more, that's great. Conversely, even 10 minutes a day can help. Natural light even helps people to heal faster.

Health experts are now touting the benefits of "The Green Effect" and "The Blue Effect." Just 10 minutes a day of exposure to natural blue colors — such as the sky and bodies of water — ponds, lakes, rivers, streams, and creeks have very positive effects on our health. So does exposure to green — such as natural grass, fields, herbs, plants, and mountains. Today take a look at your schedule and decide where and when you can fit more outdoor time in.

People in the Mediterranean region look for any excuse to be outside – from strolling to eating, talking and exercising "outdoors" is the preferred place to be. Even if you live in a cold environment, bundling up and spending time outdoors, preferably with a bit of sun exposure is worth the effort.

Check out the following Schedule Base Template.

Day Four — Focus on quality of sleep

Sleep is one of the most overlooked contributors to our overall well-being. If you want to enjoy optimal health, making sleep a priority is a necessity. Adequate quality sleep can help you to metabolize and digest food better, improve digestion, reduce food cravings, improve mood, maintain a healthy weight. Chapters 11 and 13 discuss the importance of sleep and obstacles to get a solid seven-hours' worth of good sleep per night in greater detail. If you're not currently getting enough sleep, take a look at those chapters and consider speaking with your healthcare provider.

Napping is good for physical and mental health. It can help us to rejuvenate and restart. Taken after lunch, siesta-style naps — even as short as 10-25 minutes — can help you to avoid afternoon slumps, balance hormones, improve overall sleep time, reduce the risk of a cardiovascular event, lose weight, as well as increase productivity and libido.

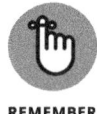

REMEMBER

When you think about the areas of your health that you have positive influence over, diet and exercise play the largest role. Sleep sets the stage for the diet and exercise to work.

If you can't nap during the day at work, indulge in them on your days off. During the work week try a short mediation or breath work after lunch to give your brain a break from all the thinking. Be sure to schedule these into your daily activities.

Following is the Schedule Base Template to check out.

Day Five — Focus on looking on the bright side

A wonderful affirmation to say first thing in the morning is "I look for reasons to feel good and I find them." Make it your life's work to look for things to feel good about, as these thoughts will improve your health. Today, really focus on the issues and people you are spending yourself thinking about. Do they make you feel good or bad? If the answer is "bad," then shift your attention to what feels good. As simple as this may sound, the act of "pivoting" or changing focus from something negative to something positive can be as difficult as breaking an addiction to smoking, drinking, or unhealthy eating.

The payoff for choosing to make this change daily, however, has positive effects on your health by helping you to cope with stress better and ultimately find joy (See Chapter 11). If you think about it, you always have something to be grateful for — the breath we breath, the eyes we see with, the sound of children's laughter, and so on. Modern culture sets us up to think that we can't stop worrying or thinking negatively until we purchase or achieve everything we ever wanted, but that simply isn't the case. The happier that we are in the present, the more good health and good fortune we bring to ourselves and the world. The "selfish" act of choosing to be happy despite whatever negativity is going on can help you to reverse your pre-diabetes diagnosis and enjoy better health in general.

Today make a note of any old scripts that you have in your mind. What's preventing you from true happiness? Does a perceived lack of not having enough of something — money, work, a relationship, understanding, and so forth . . . prevent you from enjoying this present moment? If so, it's time to ask yourself the following:

» Is this thought benefitting me in any way?

» If I focus on what I don't have or what I don't like, will it help me to get it?

» Would I rather be happy or right?

Many times in life you will be right about an issue and choose to hold negative thoughts and beliefs about them based on principle. But the truth of the matter is that those negative thoughts and feelings are only harming you, the benign issues and other parties don't feel them. If you're reading this book, it's because you want to improve your health or the health of someone that you care about. You owe it to yourself and them to feel your best.

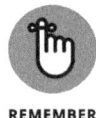

REMEMBER

From today on, when you think about negative situations, ask for ways to see them in a different light and for help focusing on something positive. Create a list of things that you love thinking about — no matter how seemingly insignificant or silly — it could be the waves of the ocean, or birds, or butterflies — anything that makes you smile unconditionally. Whenever you catch yourself focusing on the negative — make the decision to choose the bright side where your health and happiness live and focus your attention there.

Some of you may be thinking that all of this sounds a bit Pollyannaish or that it's wishful thinking. But there is science-based evidence that you get what you focus on, so it's better to focus on what you want. When people think of the Mediterranean region, they may think of fancy ports with yachts or idyllic vacations, but the truth of the matter is that people in this part of the world have survived everything from wars to famine to draughts and everything in between. Catastrophes and disasters big and small have been taking place in the Mediterranean region for millennia. Because of that, the local attitude is that the present moment is precious. When given the decision, most people choose to look on the bright side and create their own happiness as often as possible. This is another reason why they have enjoyed such good health for so long, and you can do the same.

Check out the following Schedule Base Template.

Day 6 — Focus on pleasurable activity

Did you know that while all activity can be beneficial, doing the ones which we enjoy the most can help to keep our minds, bodies, and spirits the healthiest?

According to research, its in our best interest to do more of what we love — regardless of what it is. Do you have a hobby or pastime that gets you out of your head and makes you feel good? It doesn't matter if it's running, gardening, biking, dancing, writing poetry, sewing, painting, or drawing. The act of physically doing something (as opposed to watching something on TV or scrolling — even though there's time for that too) can help to reduce stress, broaden your social circle, lift spirits, reduce chronic pain, and improve your quality of life.

Today look for ways to do more of what you love more often. We give you bonus points for doing those ideas outside and with others when possible.

Follow the Schedule Base Template in the next section.

Day 7 — Focus on relaxation and relationships

Today's activity is meant to be practiced on your day of rest. Italians have the concept of *dolce far niente* which means "the sweetness of doing nothing." Nowadays you see people promoting this concept on social media while drinking or eating. But the idea behind it is really that you dedicate a certain amount of time for yourself per week when you literally don't have anything to do. No reading, screen time, activities, and so on. You can just sit or lay down and relax — perhaps at the beach or outdoors. Even doing this at home can give your brain, body, and emotions some waking hours when they can reset and simply "be" without any pressure. Decide when and how to fit a few hours or a full day of this into your schedule.

A day of rest is also a great time to spend quality time with loved ones. Consider seeing a friend or spending quality time with loved ones. Even a phone or video call can help you to feel connected and prepare you emotionally for the week ahead.

Check out the Schedule Base Template here.

Schedule Base Template Days 1-7 — Wake up

Give thanks/prayer — start your day on a positive note whichever way works for you.

>> **Get Out of Bed**

- Freshening up — shower, bath, and so on.

- Sun exposure — open the windows and blinds and let the sunlight in. If it's cold outside — still open a window to let fresh air in.

» **Pre-Breakfast**

- Gratitude — Make a gratitude list and give sincere thanks for everything that you have.
- Meditate or do breath work.
- Prep/cook breakfast.

» **Eat Breakfast**

- See the recipes in Chapter 15.
- Housework, landscaping, gardening, and so on.

» **Work**

- Snack — See the suggestions in Chapter 15.
- Lunch — Use this as a time to catch up with friends/colleagues.
- Exercise — Take a walk around the building or to or from the café.
- Invite someone to dinner or make plans to have a "virtual" dinner with someone if you live alone.

» **Work**

- Cook dinner.

» **Dinner**

- Go for an evening stroll or exercise — preferably with friends.

» **Evening Activities**

- Socialize — use this time to catch up with other friends.
- Plan next day's meals.

» **Before Bed**

- Read.
- Bath or shower.
- Calming Tisane (herbal beverages).

A LIFESTYLE THAT REDUCES INFLAMMATION

A positive/grateful mindset paired with the proper diet and exercise can help balance the negative effects of some genetic patterns and exposure to environmental factors and toxins that may result in inflammation in the body. Acute inflammation on the surface of the body manifests itself as redness, heat, swelling, and pain and is usually a temporary and useful response to damage or a threat from external factors that should naturally resolve and heal. But when inflammation persists, is misdirected, or is triggered by recurring harmful factors, it damages the cells in the body and may become chronic and result in serious illnesses, blood clots, and cancers.

Chronic inflammation can be driven by a number of factors, including smoking, environmental toxins, a poor-quality diet, and a persistent state of what is called *oxidative stress* — when the chemistry of cells is out of balance, when atoms or molecules called *free radicals* aren't controlled. Free radicals, either from environment or by-products from metabolic processes, are highly reactive and can cause damage to structures in the body through a process called *oxidation* — a chemical reaction that involves them taking electrons from other stable molecules. This outcome can result in a destructive chain reaction and further damage to cell structures and can cause an inflammatory response. If this isn't counterbalanced by internal healing processes, supported by antioxidant compounds found in the healthy ingredients of diet, then chronic inflammation can occur.

Extra-virgin olive oil, garlic, chilies, fish, tomatoes, green leafy vegetables, green tea, berries, and cherries are all anti-inflammatory foods because they're rich in antioxidant compounds such as polyphenols. Eating combinations of these delicious ingredients, along with avoiding foods fried in unhealthy oils, large amounts of red or fatty meat, processed foods, excess alcohol, and simple carbohydrates and sugars from processed bread and pasta can have major health benefits. Diets high in saturated fats, sugar, and an excess of polyunsaturated omega-6 fats from vegetable oils are *pro-inflammatory* — they increase levels of inflammation in the body in contrast to those foods that suppress and control chronic inflammation.

5

Avoiding or Reversing Prediabetes

Chapter **15**

Cooking and Eating for Health and Enjoyment

L earning to cook and eat with both pleasure and health in mind is integral to enjoying life and good health at the same time.

In this chapter, you will learn how to combine ingredients and prepare meals and snacks to keep your blood sugar in order and prevent you from developing Type 2 diabetes.

Learning to Cook for Health and Enjoyment

If you're reading this book, then perhaps either you or someone you care for has been diagnosed with prediabetes. Speaking from experience, we know that embarking on the task of "having" to cook diabetes–friendly meals can be daunting to say the least. Chef Amy learned to create meals that would prevent blood sugar from spiking while satisfying her family's palates when she was only 15 years old. If she can do it, so can you.

Obviously, not everyone loves cooking. When Chef Amy was told that she needed to cook diabetes-friendly meals to comply with her mother's then new diagnosis was not happy. Nowadays she's a professional chef and cookbook author, but as a teenager, the task of putting dinner on the table at night and making it healthy was not her idea of fun. Sure, she loved baking with her grandmothers and making special occasion dishes, but those didn't require nutritional consideration. She felt like her new "chore" of cooking for her mom (and the rest of her family) with healthy recipes was a form of punishment.

When you're told that you must eat a certain way that deviates from what you're used to, it can feel very disheartening, to say the least. You may have to give up some of your favorite foods or cooking styles. Planning ahead becomes a necessity, and you have to really get creative with nutritious ingredients.

I remember a turning point in my personal story. After a few weeks of begrudgingly making dinner with new recipes, at one point, I remember thinking, "you're going to have to do this anyway, so you may as well make it as fun as possible." After being forced to make healthier and more nutritiously conscious meals, Chef Amy began challenging herself to make the best tasting, most nutritious combinations possible with whatever ingredients she had on hand. Fast forward 3 decades, and that's still her philosophy today.

Even if you don't love cooking already, there's still time to embrace the activity. Home cooked food offers many more nutritional benefits than processed or store-bought foods. If you enjoy making the foods that are good for you, you'll also benefit from the mood boosting effects of doing what you love.

The recipes in this chapter equip you with breakfast, snack, lunch, and dinner recipes that are rich in health-boosting properties and offer glucose balancing solutions for every meal of the day.

Breakfasts

Breakfast conjures up different images for different people, and most have very strong opinions about it. Some love it, others hate it. With the popularity of intermittent fasting some people have sworn off breakfast altogether. Unless your doctor has recommended fasting, however, those with prediabetes should generally enjoy regular meals to prevent blood sugar spikes. It's recommended that those with prediabetes or diabetes should eat a balanced meal within the first few hours of waking.

The notion of what constitutes breakfast is also very debatable. Cultural styles and personal preferences set the tone for the way most people eat in the morning. Breakfast foods can consist of everything from a donut or bagel and coffee to beans, eggs, meat, and cheese, to even fish, seafood soups, and mushrooms depending on where you live and how you're raised.

For this reason, when embarking on a healthful eating plan that will help you feel your best while enjoying yourself in the process, it's best to consider a few things when deciding what to eat for breakfast and other meals.

If you have prediabetes or diabetes, you should determine the following before enjoying a specific breakfast (or meal in general):

>> Is this item/dish/meal balanced in macronutrients? (Does it contain a healthful fat, good source of protein, and quality carbohydrates)?

>> Do I enjoy eating this type of food? (Some people like protein shakes in the morning, others like hot breakfasts, etc.).

>> How can I fit this recipe into my lifestyle? (Do you need to focus on "make ahead" dishes, quick assembly meals, can you dedicate a few hours on your day off to prepping, etc.?).

>> Does this dish contain ingredients that are known to be beneficial for people with diabetes (Polyphenol rich fresh fruit, vegetables, and extra virgin olive oil, healthful fats like those found in almonds and fish, omega-3's in seafood, fiber found in whole grains and vegetables, etc.?).

The recipes included in this section offer a base for different types of breakfasts that can be easily incorporated into a busy life. Recipes in this chapter include:

- **Mixed Oatmeal and Berries with Cinnamon and Almonds**

Can be prepped the night before and eaten on the go — if needed.

- **Citrus Yogurt Bowl with Sweet Spices and Flax Seeds**

Can be prepared in a few minutes or in advance — is portable and can also be enjoyed as a snack.

- **Savory Mediterranean Breakfast Platter**

Can be prepared the night before — is portable and can also do double duty as a portable lunch or dinner.

- **Chocolate Almond Waffles with Warm Berry Compote**

This recipe takes a bit longer to prepare and allows you to indulge in classic weekend breakfast flavors whenever the time permits.

- **Avocado Toast with Scrambled Eggs**

Make this delicious and satisfying toast when you have time to sit down and enjoy breakfast. This recipe can also do double duty as lunch or dinner.

Oatmeal and Mixed Berries with Cinnamon and Almonds

PREP TIME: 5 MIN	COOK TIME: 25 MIN	YIELD: 4 SERVINGS

INGREDIENTS

1 cup (176g) steel oats

1 teaspoon (3g) ground pure (Ceylon) cinnamon

½ cup (71g) whole raw almonds, chopped and toasted (see Note)

2 teaspoons (2g) raw honey* See Note

2 cups (296g) mixed fresh blueberries, raspberries, and strawberries

1 cup (100g) unsweetened almond milk* See Note

DIRECTIONS

1 In a medium saucepan bring 3 cups (720mL) water to a boil over high heat. Stir in the oats.

2 Reduce the heat to medium and cook for 10 minutes. Add in the cinnamon, and almonds, and cook for 10-15 more minutes, stirring occasionally, until oatmeal is tender.

3 Stir in the berries and raw honey and place into 4 individual bowls. Drizzle ¼ cup (68mL) almond milk over each bowl and additional cinnamon over the top (if desired). Serve warm or allow to cool to room temperature and store in the refrigerator until serving.

PER SERVING: *Calories 325 (From Fat 109); Fat 12g (Saturated 1g); Cholesterol 0mg; Sodium 1mg; Carbohydrate 47g (Dietary Fiber 10g); Protein 5g.*

NOTE: Raw honey is unheated and unfiltered and still contains natural antioxidants and enzymes that are beneficial to the health. Almond milk comes in many forms. Always look for unsweetened almond milk with the shortest ingredient list possible — almonds and water is ideal.

To toast almonds, place them on a lined baking sheet and place into a 400°F degree oven for 5-10 minutes until they begin to release their aroma and turn color. This can be done up to a week in advance and almonds can be stored in the refrigerator.

TIP: Keep cooked oatmeal (without the fruit) on hand for busy mornings. Add in berries, apples, or diced fruit of your choice before eating.

VARY IT! While steel oats offer the most nutrition, you can substitute old-fashioned oats to save time in a pinch. Add in ¼ cup (22g) dark cocoa to make chocolate oatmeal, if desired.

Citrus Yogurt Bowl with Sweet Spices and Flax Seeds

PREP TIME: 5 MIN	COOK TIME: 0 MIN	YIELD: 2 SERVINGS

INGREDIENTS

4 mandarin oranges, zested

½ cup (113g) organic plain (unsweetened) Greek yogurt

2 tablespoons (14g) grounded/milled flax seeds

2 tablespoons (18g) sesame seeds

½ cup (71g) whole, unroasted almonds

1 teaspoon (7g) raw honey

1 teaspoon (3g) ground pure (Ceylon) cinnamon

½ teaspoon (1g) ground cardamom

¼ teaspoon (.5g) ground cloves

DIRECTIONS

1 Peel the oranges and divide into segments. Place ½ of the segments in 2 bowls.

2 Spoon ¼ cup (57g) yogurt into each bowl.

3 Scatter 1 tablespoon (7g) flax seeds, 1 tablespoon (9g) sesame seeds and ½ of the honey and almonds over each bowl. Top with remaining orange segments and orange zest.

4 Sprinkle cinnamon, cardamom, and cloves over the top of each and serve.

PER SERVING: *Calories 465 (From Fat 234); Fat 25g (Saturated 2g); Cholesterol 6mg; Sodium 53mg; Carbohydrate 41g (Dietary Fiber 11g); Protein 25g.*

TIP: Make this recipe overnight for a creamier consistency.

NOTE: Flaxseed was cultivated in Babylon as early as 3000 BCE and contains a high amount of omega-3 fatty acids, which can help lower cholesterol and improve the complexion. The Greek yogurt in this recipe provides additional benefit of inulin, a compound which helps to balance blood sugar levels naturally.

VARY IT! You can put the same ingredients and a handful of ice in the blender and blend until smooth for delicious smoothies that also make great post workout snacks. Swap out orange segments for fresh berries, if desired.

Savory Mediterranean Breakfast Platter

PREP TIME: 5 MIN	COOK TIME: 0 MIN	YIELD: X2 SERVINGS

INGREDIENTS

2 Persian cucumbers or

1 English cucumber, sliced

2 Roma tomatoes, sliced

1 handful fresh mint or parsley, or a combination of both, cleaned

1 cup (227g) plain Greek yogurt

2 hardboiled eggs

2 tablespoons (27g) Amy Riolo Selections or other good-quality extra virgin olive oil

2 teaspoons (3g) Za'atar spice mix,

or unrefined sea salt

1 slice whole wheat pita, cut into quarters

DIRECTIONS

1 On two separate plates or a large platter, arrange cucumber slices and tomatoes in a decorative pattern on half of the plate.

2 Add fresh mint and/or parsley to the center of the plate.

3 Dollop Greek yogurt on one quadrant of the plate.

4 Slice the hardboiled eggs into quarters and place next to the labneh.

5 Drizzle the egg and yogurt with olive oil and sprinkle with Za'atar or sea salt. Serve with whole wheat pita quarters.

PER SERVING: *Calories 446 (From Fat 191); Fat 21g (Saturated 4g); Cholesterol 224mg; Sodium 346mg; Carbohydrate 29g (Dietary Fiber 4g); Protein 36g.*

TIP: This quick and nutritious Mediterranean power plate can be a great portable lunch, snack or dinner as well.

NOTE: Za'atar is a wild thyme spice mix that hails from the Middle East. It usually contains sumac, sea salt, coriander, and sesame seeds. If you can't find it, substitute your favorite spice or unrefined sea salt.

VARY IT! Use a combination of your own favorite vegetables and cook the egg in a different way if you choose.

Chocolate Almond Waffles with Warm Berry Compote

PREP TIME: 5 MIN	COOK TIME: 10 MIN	YIELD: 2 SERVINGS

INGREDIENTS

1 large egg

2 teaspoons (8g) pure vanilla extract

¼ cup (25g) organic milk or almond milk

1 Tablespoon (7g) milled/ground flax seeds

2 Tablespoons (11g) cocoa powder

1 cup (112g) almond flour

Pinch salt

½ teaspoon (2g) baking soda

1 cup (148g) fresh blueberries and sliced strawberries. Divided

1 teaspoon (3g) Ceylon cinnamon

1 tablespoon (21g) good quality raw honey

1 teaspoon (5g) EVOO, for waffle maker

DIRECTIONS

1 Plug in the waffle maker (see TIP below).

2 In a medium bowl, whisk together the egg vanilla, and milk.

3 Stir in the flax seeds, cocoa powder, flour, salt, and baking soda, mixing well to combine.

4 If the batter seems to thick, add water, a tablespoon at a time to make a batter the consistency of a slightly thicker than normal pancake batter.

5 Place the ¾ of the blueberries and strawberries, the cinnamon, and the honey in a blender or food processor and puree until smooth.

6 Pour the berry juice into a small saucepan, bring to a simmer, and remove from heat.

7 Brush the waffle maker with the oil. Pour approximately ⅓ cup (80mL) of batter onto 2 quadrants of the hot maker.

8 Using a spoon, spread the batter to the corners before shutting the lid.

9 Cook until waffles are puffy and golden (approximately 3-5 minutes). Some waffle makers will have lights to tell you when the iron is preheated and when the waffles have finished cooking.

10 Spoon remaining berries and berry syrup over the warm waffles and serve immediately.

PER SERVING: *Calories 504 (From Fat 320); Fat 36g (Saturated 4g); Cholesterol 106mg; Sodium 432mg; Carbohydrate 38g (Dietary Fiber 12g); Protein 18g.*

TIP: Waffle makers vary from manufacturer to manufacturer, so it is a good idea to test yours out- both to find out exactly how much batter you need to make the proper-sized waffle on your iron, and to test the amount of time it takes to accurately cook the waffles.

NOTE: This recipe makes a nutritious and decadent breakfast perfect for weekends and special occasions. Try making extra waffles and freezing them in airtight plastic bags to use at another time.

VARY IT! By swapping out the baking soda in this recipe for baking powder, you can create gluten-free pancakes instead of waffles. Swap out raspberries for others if desired.

Avocado Toast with Scrambled Eggs

| PREP TIME: 5 MIN | COOK TIME: 6 MIN | YIELD: 4 SERVINGS |

INGREDIENTS

4 slices good quality whole wheat, barley, or oat bread

4 teaspoons (18g) Amy Riolo Selections or other good quality extra virgin olive oil, divided

2 ripe avocados, halved and pitted (see Figure 15-1)

⅛ teaspoon (.6g) unrefined sea salt or fleur de sel, plus extra for sprinkling

4 teaspoons (10g) flax seeds

½ cup cherry (75g) tomatoes, diced and divided

4 large eggs

Freshly ground black pepper

½ cup (75g) cherry tomatoes, diced

1 cup (30g) microgreens, baby spinach, baby kale, or baby arugula

DIRECTIONS

1 Toast the bread in a toaster or under the broiler to desired doneness.

2 Drizzle ½ teaspoon (5g) of EVOO over each piece of bread.

3 Scoop the avocado out of the shell, and place the flesh from ½ of each avocado on each of the pieces of bread.

4 Drizzle 1 teaspoon (5g) EVOO over the toast pieces (1/4 teaspoon (1g) each).

5 Sprinkle sea salt and scatter flax seeds over the top.

6 Combine eggs in a small bowl, add in ¼ cup (60mL) water, and whisk until frothy. Season with ¼ teaspoon (1g) sea salt and freshly ground pepper to taste.

7 Heat remaining teaspoon EVOO in a skillet over medium heat. Add egg mixture and cook, stirring with a spatula, until cooked through. Fold in ½ of cherry tomatoes.

8 Top toasts with eggs and remaining 1/2 tomato pieces and ¼ cup (7g) of mixed greens or baby spinach, kale, or arugula. Serve hot.

PER SERVING: *Calories 622 (From Fat 387); Fat 43g (Saturated 8g); Cholesterol 423mg; Sodium 548mg; Carbohydrate 40g (Dietary Fiber 16g); Protein 25g.*

TIP: It can be difficult to buy ripe avocados in many non-tropical climates. In supermarkets they are often either all ready at the same time, or hard at the time of purchase. If they are hard, leave them at room temperature until ripe. If they are all ripe at time of purchase, peel, pit and remove the flesh. Mash the flesh with a bit of lemon or lime juice. Mix well and place in an airtight container until using.

NOTE: Avocados are so creamy and decadent, that it is hard to believe that they are good for us. They are full of vitamins, nutrients, and heart-healthy fats, while also being cholesterol free. It is believed that adding avocado to the diet may help those with diabetes to lose weight and increase insulin sensitivity while lowering cholesterol.

VARY IT! Sauteed spinach, kale, collards, Swiss chard, or any other green could be used instead of avocado.

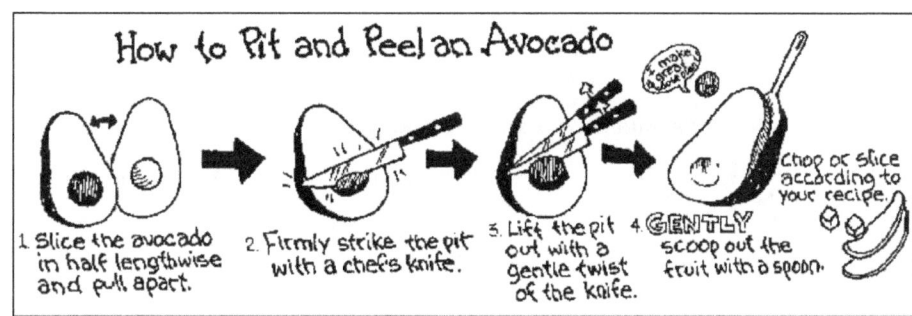

FIGURE 15-1:
Pitting an avocado the easy way.

Snacks

There is a misconception that people who are diagnosed with diabetes or prediabetes eat too much. Many times, however, it's just the opposite. Skipping meals, eating the wrong kinds of food, and not eating enough can wreak havoc on your blood sugar levels. People diagnosed with prediabetes shouldn't go more than 5 hours without eating a balanced meal or snack.

Be sure to plan ahead and have snacks readily available while you are home, traveling, or working so that you can regulate your blood sugar levels.

Recipes included in this chapter are:

» **Blueberry Banana Smoothie** — can also be enjoyed at breakfast

Creamy Homemade Hummus & Crudites — can also be a light lunch or dinner

Tzatziki Sauce and Whole Wheat Pita Chips — can do double duty at breakfast or lunch

Date and Dark Chocolate Energy Bites — Also a healthful dessert

Kale, Apple, and Citrus Salad with Walnuts and Creamy Herb Dressing — Add more of your favorite protein to turn this into a complete meal

Each of these recipes contains all three macronutrients — healthful fats, quality protein and carbs which when combined can prevent blood sugar from spiking. In addition, they contain powerful bioactive compounds called polyphenols which are effective in reducing inflammation and boosting health benefits. Keep them on hand to enjoy as needed.

Blueberry Banana Smoothie

INGREDIENTS

1 cup (148g) blueberries

1 ripe banana, sliced

1 cup (227g) Full fat Plain Greek Yogurt

½ cup (109g) ice

1 tsp (4g) pure vanilla extract

½ cup (48g) ground almonds

DIRECTIONS

1 Place all ingredients into a blender and blend on high power until smooth and creamy.

2 Pour into 2 glasses and serve cold.

PER SERVING: Calories 380 (From Fat 119); Fat 13g (Saturated 1g); Cholesterol 12mg; Sodium 93mg; Carbohydrate 37g (Dietary Fiber 6g); Protein 32g.

TIP: Keep ripe bananas in the freezer to create this sweet, frothy smoothie when needed.

NOTE: This smoothie is also great pre or post workouts or to keep blood sugar from spiking in between meals as a snack.

VARY IT! Any fresh fruit — pomegranate seeds, berries, avocados, oranges, or a combination can be used in place of blueberries in this recipe. You can also keep frozen fruit in the freezer specifically for the purpose of making smoothies — this also eliminates the need for ice.

Creamy Homemade Hummus & Crudites

PREP TIME: 10 MIN	COOK TIME: 0 MIN	YIELD: 4 SERVINGS

INGREDIENTS

1 cup (164g) cooked or no salt added canned chickpeas, drained and rinsed

1 garlic clove, minced

⅓ cup (75g) tahini (sesame puree)

3 teaspoons (40g) Amy Riolo Selections, or other good quality extra virgin olive oil, divided

½ teaspoon (3g) salt

2 ice cubes

Dash of paprika, for garnish

1 cup (91g) broccoli flowerets, for serving

1 cup (100g) cauliflower flowerets, for serving

4 celery stalks, cut in half and quartered, for serving

1 English cucumber, sliced, for serving

DIRECTIONS

1 Peel chickpeas and place them in a food processor, reserving a few for garnish.

2 Add the garlic, tahini, 2 tablespoons olive oil, and salt, to the food processor. Puree until smooth.

3 Add the ice cubes and continue to puree.

4 If hummus isn't creamy enough, add water, tablespoon by tablespoon, to get an extra creamy consistency (you should need less than ¼ cup (60mL) in total).

5 Scrape down the sides of the food processor, and puree for 1 to 2 additional minutes. Taste and adjust seasonings if necessary.

6 Spoon onto a small round dish. Using the back of a spoon, make dents in the top and fill the dents with remaining tablespoon of olive oil.

7 Sprinkle paprika and arrange remaining chickpeas on the top. Serve with crudites.

PER SERVING: *Calories 295 (From Fat 185); Fat 21g (Saturated 3g); Cholesterol 0mg; Sodium 425mg; Carbohydrate 22g (Dietary Fiber 7g); Protein 9g.*

TIP: If not serving immediately, store hummus in a container with a lid in the refrigerator.

NOTE: In the Eastern Mediterranean countries, hummus can be served with slices of meat or chicken on top. If you have leftover meat, this is a great way to make a full meal out of it.

VARY IT! You can make a delicious, nutritious, and creamy puree out of all kinds of beans and lentils. Just don't call it hummus! /The word means "chickpea" in Arabic.

Tzatziki Sauce with Whole Wheat Pita Chips

PREP TIME: 10 MIN	COOK TIME: 2 MIN	YIELD: 4 SERVINGS

INGREDIENTS

2 pieces of whole wheat pita, cut into pieces

3 tablespoons (41g) Amy Riolo Selections Extra Virgin Olive Oil, divided

2 organic English cucumbers, peeled and shredded

¼ teaspoon (.3g) unrefined sea salt

3 cups (680g) plain, low-fat Greek organic yogurt, preferably made from sheep and goat's milk, if possible

¼ cup (2g) fresh dill or mint, chopped

1 garlic clove, minced

1 small yellow onion, grated and drained

DIRECTIONS

1 Preheat broiler. Place pita on a baking sheet, drizzle with 2 Tablespoons (26g) EVOO, and toss to coat. Broil for a minute or two until toasted. Remove from oven.

2 Place cucumbers in a colander and press out water with a fork.

3 Spoon the cucumbers into a medium sized bowl and stir in the yogurt.

4 Stir in dill or mint, garlic, and onion.

5 Add garlic and onion and stir.

6 Spoon onto a shallow dish and smooth out with the back of a spoon. Drizzle with remaining tablespoon (13g) of EVOO. Serve with pita chips.

PER SERVING: *Calories 388 (From Fat 110); Fat 12g (Saturated 2g); Cholesterol 19mg; Sodium 250mg; Carbohydrate 29g (Dietary Fiber 2g); Protein 41g.*

TIP: If you can't find English cucumbers, Persian cucumbers work well in this recipe too. If you must use conventional American cucumbers, remove the seeds before making this dip.

NOTE: This classic combination is one of the healthiest dishes possible due to the antioxidants, minerals, and vitamins in the cucumbers, macro-nutrients and inulin (a compound that helps keep blood sugar balanced) and probiotics in the yogurt, anti-inflammatory aspects of the garlic, onion, and extra virgin olive oil combine to make a mouthwatering and nutritious recipe. Use this as a dip or a sauce for grilled chicken and meat. In the summertime, it makes a cool and creamy breakfast.

VARY IT! Serve Tzatziki with crudites instead of pita chips or use it as a "bed" to serve grilled chicken or fish on. Place this mixture in the blender and puree until smooth. Refrigerate overnight for a cold soup.

Date and Dark Chocolate Energy Bites

PREP TIME: 10 MIN	COOK TIME: 0 MIN	YIELD: 6 SERVINGS

INGREDIENTS

1 pound (454g) soft dates, pitted

¼ cup (43g) dark chocolate (85% or higher) pieces

2 Tablespoons (27g) Amy Riolo Selections, or other good quality extra virgin olive oil

½ pound (227g) blanched almonds

1 teaspoon (4g) vanilla extract

½ teaspoon (1g) ground cinnamon

3 Tablespoons (16g) raw dark cocoa powder, if desired

DIRECTIONS

1 Place dates, chocolate, EVOO, ¼ cup (60mL) water, almonds, vanilla, and cinnamon in a food processor.

2 Pulse to form a smooth paste. Shape dough into date-size balls.

3 Roll date balls into cocoa powder coat, if desired. Arrange on a serving platter. Store extras in the fridge for up to a week.

PER SERVING: *Calories 520 (From Fat 244); Fat 27g (Saturated 4g); Cholesterol 0mg; Sodium 13mg; Carbohydrate 69g (Dietary Fiber 11g); Protein 11g.*

TIP: Keep these on hand for a quick snack in between meals or as a post workout treat.

NOTE: Choose the softest dates possible — Such as Medjool for this recipe.

VARY IT! Even a few dates and a handful of raw almonds alone make a great snack on the go.

Kale, Apple, and Citrus Salad with Walnuts and Creamy Herb Dressing

PREP TIME: 20 MIN	COOK TIME: 15 MIN	YIELD: 2 SERVINGS

INGREDIENTS

1 pound (454g) fresh baby kale

½ cup (50g) unsalted walnuts, chopped

2 apples, diced

2 carrots, peeled and shredded

¼ cup (54g) Amy Riolo Selections or other good quality extra virgin olive oil

Juice and zest of 1 orange

Juice and zest of 1 lemon

2 Tablespoons (11g) freshly chopped mint

2 Tablespoons (11g) freshly chopped parsley

1 tsp (7g) raw honey

⅛ tsp (.6g) unrefined sea salt

¼ tsp (.5g) freshly ground black pepper

DIRECTIONS

1 Place kale, walnuts, apples, in a large bowl.

2 In a medium bowl, whisk together the EVOO, orange and lemon juice and zest, mint, parsley, honey, salt and pepper until creamy and emulsified.

3 When it is time to serve the salad, drizzle the vinaigrette over the top and toss to coat.

PER SERVING: *Calories 657 (From Fat 408); Fat 45g (Saturated 6g); Cholesterol 0mg; Sodium 260mg; Carbohydrate 63g (Dietary Fiber 11g); Protein 13g.*

TIP: If you have leftover grilled meat, chicken, fish, or hard boiled eggs you can add them to this salad.

NOTE: Soft goat cheese is also a nice addition to this salad, if desired.

VARY IT! Swap out kale for spinach, collards, or arugula in this salad.

Mains

Choosing delicious and healthful main dishes are one of the keys to success for those diagnosed with prediabetes. Eating bland foods just because they're deemed good for you will only make it easier for your eating plan to be derailed. It's important to choose recipes that contain a serving of high quality carbs such as those found in whole grains, beans, legumes, and root vegetables along with healthful fats such as those found in extra virgin olive oil, avocados, nuts, and fatty fish like salmon, tuna, and swordfish. Combining those with a single serving of protein such as eggs, chicken, fish, or plant-based proteins such as legumes will give you the most bang for your buck in terms of a complete meal.

Try basing your meals around seasonal produce. Including leafy greens at lunch and dinner is always a good idea, because they're full of fiber, minerals, and anti-oxidants. Adding in lots of fresh herbs, spices, vinegar, and citrus juice will boost both the flavor and nutrient components of your meals. The recipes in this chapter pull from different global styles and taste profiles to prove that diabetes-friendly food can be as delicious as it is good for you.

Be sure to prepare extra quantities of these dishes so that you can enjoy the left-overs for lunch or freeze them for a quick dinner solution at another time:

>> **Italian Barley, Bean, and 6 Vegetable Minestrone**

Spinach, Blueberry, and Feta Salad with Herb-Roasted Chicken

Quinoa and Black Bean Burgers with Mixed Greens

Whole Wheat Pasta with Creamy Lentil Sauce and Pecorino Cheese

Grilled Citrus Marinated Salmon with Broccoli and Tzatziki Sauce

Sweet Potato, Black Bean, Avocado, and Quinoa Bowl

Roasted Fish and Mediterranean Vegetables with Barley

Creamy Chickpea Soup with Sizzling Rosemary Scented Shrimp

Nicoise Salad

Lemon and Oregano Sheet Pan Chicken and Roasted Vegetables

Use these recipes as a template and a starting place for cooking meals with pre-diabetes in mind. Once you have the hang of how they're made and the types of ingredients used you can easily swap out your favorites and what you have on hand to come up with your own mouthwatering creations.

Italian Barley, Bean, and 6 Vegetable Minestrone

PREP TIME: 15 MIN	COOK TIME: 1 HOUR 10 MINS	YIELD: 4 SERVINGS

INGREDIENTS

¼ cup (54g) plus 1 tablespoon (14g) Amy Riolo Selections or other good quality extra virgin olive oil

1 medium yellow onion, finely chopped

2 carrots, finely chopped

1 celery stock, finely chopped

¼ cup (15g) flat-leaf parsley, chopped

3 garlic cloves, chopped

1 cup (70g) shredded cabbage

1 Yukon gold potato, peeled and chopped into bite-size pieces

6 cups (1.4L) homemade vegetable stock (see Chapter 8) or water

1 bay leaf

1 cup (200g) pearl barley, rinsed

2 zucchini, chopped into bite-size pieces

2 large tomatoes, chopped

½ pound (227g) string beans, chopped into bite-size pieces

1 cup (260g) cooked cannellini beans or canned cannellini beans, drained and rinsed

DIRECTIONS

1 Heat 1 Tablespoon (14g) olive oil in a large stockpot over medium heat.

2 Add onion, carrot, and celery, and stir. Sauté for 3 to 5 minutes or until tender.

3 Add parsley and garlic and cook for 1 minute longer.

4 Stir in cabbage and potato. Pour in stock or water, add bay leaf and barley increase heat to high, and bring to a boil. Reduce heat to medium–low and simmer, covered for 30 minutes.

5 Increase heat to high and stir in zucchini, tomatoes, string beans, and cannellini beans. Reduce heat to low and allow to simmer, covered, for 10 minutes, or until vegetables are tender. Stir in salt and pepper.

6 When soup is finished cooking, taste, and adjust seasonings, if necessary.

7 Serve soup hot, topped with parmesan cheese and an additional Tablespoon of EVOO on each bowl.

PER SERVING: *Calories 631 (From Fat 217); Fat 24g (Saturated 5g); Cholesterol 11mg; Sodium 532mg; Carbohydrate 78g (Dietary Fiber 19g); Protein 26g.*

TIP: Save this recipe for when you have a little bit of time to spend in the kitchen. I always double this recipe so that I can freeze some of it in individual containers for quick lunches or dinners another time. This soup will stay fresh in air tight containers in the refrigerator for up to 5 days and the freezer for a few months.

½ teaspoon (2g)
unrefined sea salt

¼ tsp (.5g) freshly ground
black pepper

½ cup (50g) freshly grated
Parmesan cheese

NOTE: *Minestra* is the Italian word for a chunky soup containing many veg-etables, grains, and legumes. The suffix *one* as in *Minestrone,* means that the soup has lot of ingredients. Use what you've got on hand in your cup-board and refrigerator to come up with your own versions. As long as you've got vegetables, beans, and stock, you can make a *minestra* anytime.

VARY IT! Switch up the vegetables according to season and add a handful of small pasta shapes, grains, or rice, and different types of beans if you'd like. You can also make a creamier minestrone by pureeing half of it in a blender and then stirring it back into the pot with the original soup.

Spinach, Blueberry, and Feta Salad with Herb-Roasted Chicken

PREP TIME: 15 MIN	COOK TIME: 90 MIN	YIELD: 4 SERVINGS

INGREDIENTS

1 whole (3.5 pound) (1588g) chicken, cleaned and rinsed well

½ cup (108g) Amy Riolo Selections or other extra virgin olive oil, divided

1 teaspoon (5g) Unrefined sea salt

¼ teaspoon (.5g) freshly ground pepper

1 head garlic, stem sliced off, left intact

1 lemon, halved

1 teaspoon (.7g) finely chopped fresh rosemary

For Salad:

1 pound (454g) Fresh Spinach

1 cup (148g) fresh blueberries

½ cup (150g) plain feta, crumbled

¼ cup (64g) Amy Riolo Selections White Balsamic Vinegar

¼ teaspoon (1g) Unrefined sea salt

⅛ teaspoon (.3g) freshly ground pepper

DIRECTIONS

1 Preheat oven to 425°F (218°C).

2 Spread 2 Tablespoons (28g) EVOO in the bottom of a roasting pan. Place chicken in roasting pan and drizzle 3 Tablespoons (42g) olive oil over the chicken, turning to make sure that both the pan and chicken are coated.

3 Season with sea salt, freshly ground pepper, and herbs by rubbing them into the top and sides of the chicken.

4 Place garlic and ½ of lemon inside the chicken cavity, and squeeze remaining juice over the chicken.

5 Bake, uncovered, for 45 minutes. Carefully (oil tends to splatter), remove chicken from the oven and baste with pan juices.

6 Return to oven to bake for another 45 minutes, or until chicken is done. (Chicken is done when clear juices run from the thickest part of the thigh after being pierced with a fork and a thermometer registers 165°F (74°C) at the thickest part.)

7 Discard garlic and lemon from the chicken cavity. Cover chicken and wait 10 minutes before carving. In a small bowl combine ¼ cup (56g) EVOO with white balsamic. Whisk together with a few pinches of sea salt and freshly ground black pepper.

8 In a large bowl combine spinach, blueberries, and feta. Toss to coat with dressing. Carve the chicken into 8 pieces and serve each with an equal portion of salad.

PER SERVING: *Calories 756 (From Fat 455); Fat 45g (Saturated 14g); Cholesterol 227mg; Sodium 1244mg; Carbohydrate 14g (Dietary Fiber 3g); Protein 58g.*

TIP: Add roasted vegetables of your choice to the sides of the pan and allow to roast the remaining 40 minutes with the chicken, if desired.

NOTE: Make the chicken a day or two in advance, if desired.

VARY IT! You can make the salad and serve it with rotisserie chicken or leftover lamb or other types of protein, if desired.

Quinoa and Black Bean Burgers with Mixed Greens

PREP TIME: 10 MIN	COOK TIME: 10 MIN	YIELD: 4 SERVINGS

INGREDIENTS

1 cup (172g) cooked black beans

1 cup (185g) cooked quinoa

¼ cup (57g) plain, full fat Greek yogurt

1 bunch fresh parsley leaves, washed, dried, and finely chopped

1 roasted red pepper, finely chopped

1 teaspoon (2g) smoked paprika

½ teaspoon (2.4g) unrefined sea salt

¼ teaspoon (.5g) freshly ground black pepper

2 Tablespoons (27g) Amy Riolo Selections or other good quality EVOO

½ pound (227g) Mixed Field Greens

4 ounces (113g) soft goat cheese

DIRECTIONS

1 Place the black beans in a food processor or small blender. Purée until smooth. Spoon into a small bowl, using a spatula to scrape everything from the bottom and sides. Add in quinoa, yogurt, parsley, red pepper, paprika, salt, and pepper.

2 Using your hands or a 1/3 cup (79mL) measure or your hands, shape the mixture into 8 equal size burgers. Place them onto a cutting board or dish.

3 In a large, wide skillet, heat the EVOO over medium high heat. Coat the bottom of the pan when warm and add the burgers, gently pressing down on each one. Cook for 3-4 minutes per side, or until browned.

4 Arrange the lettuce leaves on the bottom of a serving platter. Top with the sliders. Top the patties with an equal-sized piece of goat cheese.

PER SERVING: *Calories 315 (From Fat 148); Fat 16g (Saturated 7g); Cholesterol 23mg; Sodium 385mg; Carbohydrate 26g (Dietary Fiber 7g); Protein 17g.*

TIP: You can make the patties in advance, store them in the refrigerator, and reheat before serving. If using as an appetizer, this dish pairs well with the Citrus Marinated Salmon and Vegetable Stir Fry in the next section.

NOTE: Stuff the sliders into whole wheat pita pockets along with the lettuce to make a sandwich.

VARY IT! You can use lentils or other beans instead of black beans, if desired.

Whole Wheat Pasta with Creamy Lentil Sauce and Pecorino Cheese

PREP TIME: 10 MIN	COOK TIME: 15 MIN	YIELD: 6 SERVINGS

INGREDIENTS

1 pound (454g) whole wheat pasta

¼ teaspoon (1g) unrefined sea salt

¼ cup (54g) Amy Riolo Selections, or other good quality EVOO

1 large yellow onion, thinly sliced

2 cloves garlic, minced

1½ cups (297g) cooked brown lentils

Handful of fresh basil, chopped

1 cup (246g) whole milk ricotta cheese

¼ cup (25g) grated Pecorino cheese

1 bunch fresh parsley, finely chopped

¼ teaspoon (.5g) freshly ground black pepper

DIRECTIONS

1 Bring a large pot of water to a boil over high heat. Once it boils, add salt and cook pasta per directions or until desired doneness. Reserve ½ cup (120mL) of pasta water from cooking.

2 While pasta is cooking, add EVOO to a large wide skillet over medium high heat. Add the onion, stir to coat, and reduce heat to medium. Sauté the onion until it becomes translucent and slightly golden in color, about 10 minutes. Stir in garlic and cook for another minute.

3 Place the onions, garlic, lentils in a food processor or blender and puree until smooth. Add the pureed lentils, basil ricotta, pecorino, and parsley to a heat proof bowl. Stir in hot pasta water. Drain the pasta and place back in pot. Stir in the lentil mixture. Add freshly ground pepper and serve immediately.

PER SERVING: *Calories 508 (From Fat 152); Fat 17g (Saturated 6g); Cholesterol 24mg; Sodium 127mg; Carbohydrate 72g (Dietary Fiber 4g); Protein 22g.*

TIP: Keep caramelized or sauteed onions on hand in the refrigerator to add flavor and nutrition to meals. When possible, make the Base Recipes in Chapter 13 and keep them in the refrigerator for up to a week to use when needed.

NOTE: You can also leave the lentils whole and omit the pureeing, if desired, in this dish.

VARY IT! Make the same dish with brown rice, and/or swap the lentils for your favorite legumes.

Grilled Citrus Marinated Salmon with Broccoli and Tzatziki Sauce

PREP TIME: 15 MIN	COOK TIME: 25 MIN	YIELD: 4 SERVINGS

INGREDIENTS

2 Tablespoons (27g) Amy Riolo Selections, or other good quality EVOO

¼ cup (62g) freshly squeezed orange juice and zest

½ teaspoon (2.4g) unrefined sea salt

¼ teaspoon (.5g) freshly ground black pepper

4 salmon fillets (4 ounces each) (454g), skin on

4 cups (364g) broccoli flowerets

1 recipe Tzatziki (see recipe earlier in the chapter

DIRECTIONS

1 In a small bowl, whisk together the EVOO, orange juice, salt, and pepper together until emulsified. Place the salmon fillets in a glass baking dish and pour dressing over the top.

2 Preheat oven to 425°F (218°C). Scatter the broccoli around the sides of the salmon. Bake for 15-20 minutes until fish flakes and broccoli are tender.

3 While the fish is baking, make the Tzatziki. To serve. Place the fish on a serving platter and top with Tzatziki and orange zest. Turn broccoli to coat in pan juices and serve alongside the salmon on the plate. Serve hot.

PER SERVING: *Calories 432 (From Fat 158); Fat 18g (Saturated 5g); Cholesterol 71mg; Sodium 498mg; Carbohydrate 24g (Dietary Fiber 4g); Protein 46g.*

TIP: Prepare the broccoli and make the Yogurt sauce a day in advance for quicker prep.

NOTE: Leftovers taste great served over cooked barley or whole wheat couscous or bulgur wheat as well.

VARY IT! You can use your favorite fish, or chicken breast instead of salmon, if preferred. Replace Brussels sprouts with broccoli, cauliflower, or fennel, if prepared.

Sweet Potato, Black Bean, Avocado, and Quinoa Bowl

PREP TIME: 20 MIN	COOK TIME: 45 MIN	YIELD: 2 SERVINGS

INGREDIENTS

1 sweet potato

½ cup (85g) quinoa

2 cups (60g) fresh baby spinach

2 cups (370g) cooked
black beans

1 avocado, sliced

¼ cup (34g) unsalted cashews

4 tablespoons (54g) Amy Riolo
Selections or other good-
quality extra virgin olive oil

Juice and zest of 2 limes

1 teaspoon (7g) raw honey

⅛ teaspoon (.6g)
unrefined sea salt

¼ teaspoon (.5g) freshly ground
black pepper

DIRECTIONS

1 To cook the sweet potato, prick it with a fork and either microwave it per instructions or roast it in the oven at 425°F (218°C) for 45 minutes (or microwave if desired) or until tender.

2 Bring a cup of water to boil over high heat. Add quinoa, stir, and reduce heat to medium–low. Cook until tender (approximately 10 minutes), and then drain and allow to cool.

3 Place spinach at the bottom of two bowls or carryout containers. Top with black beans.

4 Chop sweet potato into large chunks and place on top of the spinach.

5 Scatter cooled quinoa over each. Scatter the avocado slices and cashews over the top.

6 In a medium bowl, whisk together the olive oil, lime juice, honey, salt, and pepper until creamy and emulsified.

7 When it is time to serve the salad, drizzle the vinaigrette over the top and garnish each with lime zest.

PER SERVING: *Calories 940 (From Fat 438); Fat 49g (Saturated 7g); Cholesterol 0mg; Sodium 362mg; Carbohydrate 106g (Dietary Fiber 27g); Protein 28g.*

Roasted Fish and Mediterranean Vegetables with Barley

PREP TIME: 15 MIN	COOK TIME: 50 MIN	YIELD: 6 SERVINGS

INGREDIENTS

¼ cup (54g) Amy Riolo Selections or other good quality EVOO, plus 1 teaspoon (5g), divided

2 pounds (907g) eggplant, trimmed and cut into large chunks

2 green bell peppers, sliced into rings

2 medium tomatoes, diced

3 garlic cloves, peeled and sliced

1 teaspoon (2g) Herbes de Provence or seafood seasoning

6 (4 ounces each) (113g each) fish fillets (cod, red snapper, sea bass, halibut, or your favorite)

½ teaspoon (2.4g) unrefined sea salt, divided

¼ teaspoon (.5g) freshly ground black pepper

2 lemons, 1 sliced in half, the other cut into 6 slices

1 cup (200g) pearl barley, rinsed

2 cups (480mL) homemade Vegetable Stock or water

¼ cup (15g) finely chopped fresh parsley

DIRECTIONS

1 Preheat oven to 425°F (218°C). Grease the bottom of an 11×17-inch (28×43cm) baking pan with 1 teaspoon (5g) EVOO. Cover with eggplant, pepper slices, diced tomatoes, and garlic. Sprinkle herbs over the top. Stir to combine. Place in oven and bake for 25 minutes, or until vegetables begin to soften.

2 Place the fish on top of the vegetables. Season with ¼ teaspoon (1g) salt and pepper. Drizzle the juice of the halved lemon over the top. Pour 3 tablespoons (45g) olive oil over the entire mixture. Bake for an additional 15-20 minutes, or until fish flakes easily and vegetables are cooked through.

3 Over medium heat, heat 1 tablespoon (15g) olive oil in a medium size pot with a fitted lid. Add the barley and stir to coat, stir in the remaining ¼ teaspoon (1g) salt. Add the vegetable stock and bring to a boil over high heat. Reduce heat to low, cover, and cook for 15 to 20 minutes until barley is tender. Remove from heat and stir in parsley.

4 To serve, plate fish, mix vegetables to combine and place on plate. Add barley to plates while warm and serve.

PER SERVING: *Calories 349 (From Fat 102); Fat 11g (Saturated 2g); Cholesterol 49mg; Sodium 228mg; Carbohydrate 38g (Dietary Fiber 12g); Protein 26g.*

TIP: Chop vegetables and roast them in advance, if desired, for quicker preparation.

NOTE: You can double this recipe to use the leftovers for other meals. You can make wraps, sandwiches, or even tacos using whole wheat bread and tortillas with leftovers as well.

VARY IT! Use chicken breasts or tofu instead of fish if desired.

Creamy Chickpea Soup with Sizzling Rosemary Scented Shrimp

INGREDIENTS

½ pound (227g) shrimp, peels reserved and deveined (see Figure 15-2)

1 carrot

1 onion, peeled and halved

1 rib celery

1 teaspoon (5g) unrefined sea salt

6 black peppercorns or ¼ teaspoon (.5g) ground black pepper

1 bay leaf

1 cup (200g) dried chickpeas, soaked overnight, rinsed, and drained or 3 cups (492g) cooked chickpeas

2 lemons, juiced, divided

Freshly ground black pepper, to taste

2 Tablespoons (27g) Amy Riolo Selections, or other good quality/EVOO

1 Tablespoon (2g) chopped fresh rosemary

DIRECTIONS

1 To make the shrimp stock (this can be done a day in advance): Place the shrimp peels in a large stockpot with 8 cups (2L) water, carrot, onion, and celery. Bring to a boil over high heat. Skim scum off the top of the pot and carefully discard. Add salt, peppercorns and bay leaf. Reduce heat to medium-low, simmer for 30 minutes, and strain.

2 To make the chickpea soup: Place the chickpeas in a large saucepan or stockpot with 6 cups (1.5L) of shrimp stock and onion. Bring to a boil over high heat. Reduce heat to medium-low and simmer about 1 hour or until chickpeas are tender (5 minutes if using cooked chickpeas).

3 Take off heat. Carefully place the chickpeas and the reserved liquid in the blender. Add half of the lemon juice and salt and pepper to taste. Carefully blend well until a puree is formed. Return the mixture to the pot. Taste and adjust salt if necessary. If the soup is too thick, stir in a few tablespoons of water. Stir and simmer over low heat until ready to serve.

4 To make the shrimp, heat the olive oil in a large skillet over medium high heat. When the olive oil begins to release its aroma, add the shrimp and rosemary and salt to taste. Cook for 1 to 2 minutes per side, or just until the shrimp begins to turn bright pink Drizzle with remaining lemon juice.

5 To serve, Ladle soup into 6 bowls, top with shrimp and pan juices.

PER SERVING: *Calories 224 (From Fat 65); Fat 7g (Saturated 1g); Cholesterol 57mg; Sodium 393mg; Carbohydrate 26g (Dietary Fiber 7g); Protein 15g.*

TIP: Cook the stock and chickpeas a day in advance to serve this soup in minutes on the day that you're preparing it.

NOTE: This soup recipe hails from my ancestral homeland of Calabria, Italy. Chickpeas are a good source of protein, calcium, phosphorus, potassium, and magnesium.

VARY IT! Swap out cannellini beans for chickpeas in this soup — or use leftover soup to dress whole wheat pasta.

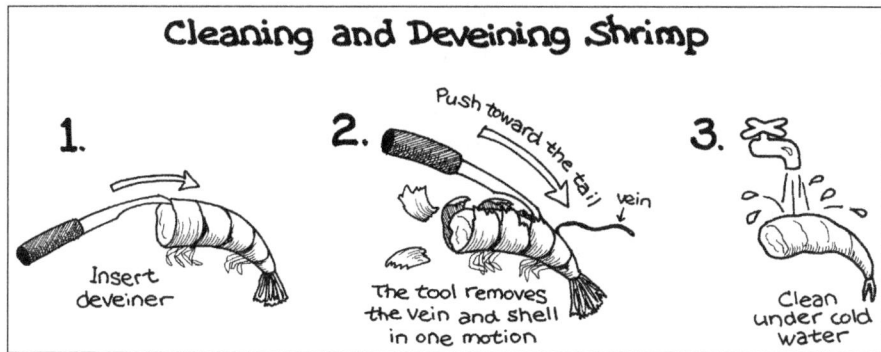

Cleaning and Deveining Shrimp

1. Insert deveiner

2. Push toward the tail — vein — The tool removes the vein and shell in one motion

3. Clean under cold water

FIGURE 15-2: Cleaning and deveining shrimp.

Nicoise Salad

| PREP TIME: 30 MIN | COOK TIME: 10 MIN | YIELD: 2 SERVINGS |

INGREDIENTS

¼ cup (54g) extra virgin olive oil

Juice of 1 lemon

2 teaspoons (2.5g) finely chopped fresh tarragon, parsley, or oregano

1 teaspoon (5g) Dijon mustard

¼ teaspoon (1g) unrefined sea salt

⅛ teaspoon (.5g) freshly ground black pepper

½ pound (227g) small young red potatoes or fingerling potatoes

4 ounces (113g) green beans, trimmed and cut into 2-inch (5cm) pieces

1 (5-ounce) (142g) cans tuna packed in water, drained, or 2 (8-ounce) (227g) grilled or otherwise cooked tuna steaks (see recipe note for cooking instructions)

2 hardboiled eggs, peeled and quartered lengthwise

1 medium head Bibb or butter lettuce, torn into bite-sized pieces

1 ripe tomato, cut into wedges

¼ cup (37g) Niçoise olives, pitted

2 tablespoons (17g) capers, rinsed well and drained

DIRECTIONS

1 Combine EVOO lemon juice, herbs, and mustard in a small bowl. Whisk well to emulsify. Season with salt and pepper and set aside.

2 Place potatoes in a large pot and cover with water. Heat on high to bring to a boil. Lower the heat medium and cook for 8 to 10 minutes or until the potatoes are fork tender. Drain. As soon as they are cool enough to handle, cut potatoes into quarters. Place them in a bowl and dress them with 2 Tablespoons of Vinaigrette.

3 Bring another pot of water to a boil. Add the green beans, reduce to medium and cook until tender but still firm to the bite, about 3–5 minutes. Drain and rinse with cold water or place in an ice bath to stop the cooking. Drain well and place in a small bowl. Dress with 1 Tablespoon Vinaigrette.

4 Arrange a bed of lettuce on a serving platter. Mound tuna in the center of lettuce. Place the tomatoes around the tuna. Arrange the potatoes and green beans in mounds at the edge of the lettuce. Arrange hardboiled eggs, olives, and capers on top in a decorative pattern. Drizzle with remaining Vinaigrette before serving.

PER SERVING: *Calories 528 (From Fat 317); Fat 35g (Saturated 6g); Cholesterol 233mg; Sodium 998mg; Carbohydrate 27g (Dietary Fiber 5g); Protein 28g.*

TIP: Cook the potatoes and green beans and make the Vinaigrette a day in advance to put this salad together quickly on a busy night or when entertaining.

NOTE: This hearty and traditional salad can be tailored to suit what your personal preferences and what you've got on hand.

VARY IT! Leftover fresh tuna steaks make a great swapout for the canned tuna when available.

Lemon and Oregano Sheet Pan Chicken and Roasted Vegetables

INGREDIENTS

¼ cup (54g) Amy Riolo Selections or other extra virgin olive oil, divided

3 pounds (1361g) chicken thighs (with skin and bone), cleaned and rinsed well

1 teaspoon (5g) Unrefined sea salt

¼ teaspoon (.5g) freshly ground pepper

1 tablespoon (3g) dried oregano, crushed

2 green bell peppers, trimmed and sliced

3 medium potatoes, cut into ¼-inch rounds

1 pint (298g) cherry tomatoes

2 cloves garlic, thinly sliced

1 lemon, halved

DIRECTIONS

1 Preheat oven to 425°F (218°C).

2 Spread 1 tablespoon (14g) EVOO in the bottom of a roasting pan. Place chicken in roasting pan and drizzle remaining 3 tablespoons (41g) olive oil over the chicken. Turn the chicken to make sure that both the pan and chicken are coated. Season with sea salt, freshly ground pepper, and oregano by rubbing them into the top and sides of the chicken. Add in peppers, potatoes, and cherry tomatoes and turn to coat.

3 Sprinkle garlic and squeeze juice over the chicken. Cover with lid or aluminum foil. Bake for 30-45 minutes, or until chicken registers 165°F on a meat thermometer. Carefully remove the lid (oil tends to splatter), remove chicken from the oven and baste with pan juices.

4 Serve warm or cool until room temperature and refrigerate to eat the next day after reheating.

PER SERVING: *Calories 693 (From Fat 374); Fat 42g (Saturated 10g); Cholesterol 166mg; Sodium 1214mg; Carbohydrate 30g (Dietary Fiber 6g); Protein 48g.*

TIP: You can also use root vegetables in this recipe in the fall, or zucchini and eggplant in the summer.

NOTE: Leftover chicken makes great soup and sandwiches.

VARY IT! Swap fish fillets for chicken thighs in this recipe and reduce the cooking time to 20-30 minutes or until fish is flaky.

Desserts

Who doesn't love dessert? Humans associate the sweet taste with safety, comfort, and nourishment because we first experience it in mother's milk. For this reason, when we eat something sweet, it truly feels like a reward. Sugar itself can be addictive, and many processed and ultra-processed package foods contain sugar and/or sugar substitutes in them to make them taste better. As a result, it's easy to develop an almost insatiable desire for sweets.

By learning to create your own tasty, sweet, and nutriously satisfying desserts, you'll be able to satisfy your sweet tooth with treats that are actually good for you. Enjoying the recipes in this chapter will help you to steer clear of the unhealthful version that can worsen your medical condition and eventually lead to full-blown diabetes diagnosis.

The recipes in this chapter include:

Dark Chocolate Berry-Studded Brownies

Almond Butter and Cinnamon "Truffles"

Chocolate Cashew Clusters

Pear, Cardamom, and Olive Oil Cake

Oatmeal and Almond Flour Cookies

By keeping healthful sweets on hand you can satisfy your sweet tooth a bit at a time when needed instead of overindulging in something which isn't good for you. Try keeping these sweet treats in the freezer, and just pulling out one a day, or when you're entertaining.

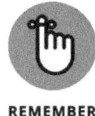

REMEMBER

If you're planning on enjoying a dessert of any type, try to eat less or skip completely the simple carbs in the meal proceeding it.

It's worth noting that each of the desserts in this chapter include healthful fat, carbs, and protein to make them balanced and prevent them from causing blood spikes. Since they do contain some simple sugars, it's best that they're enjoyed in moderation.

Dark Chocolate Berry–Studded Brownies

PREP TIME: 10 MIN	COOK TIME: 25 MIN	YIELD: 24 SERVINGS

INGREDIENTS

½ cup(108g) plus 1 teaspoon (5g) Amy Riolo Selections, or other good quality extra virgin olive oil, divided

¾ cup (94g) unbleached all-purpose flour

⅓ cup (28g) cocoa powder

1 teaspoon (5g) baking powder

½ cup (122g) unsweetened applesauce

¾ cup (144g) coconut sugar

3 large eggs

1 teaspoon (5g) cold brewed coffee or espresso

2 teaspoons (8g) vanilla extract

1 cup (170g) dark chocolate (80% or higher), cut into small pieces

1 cup (100g) coarsely chopped walnuts or pecans, divided

1 cup (123g) raspberries

DIRECTIONS

1 Heat oven to 350°F (180°C). Line an 8 × 8-inch (20 × 20cm) baking pan with parchment paper, extending over edges to form handles. Coat liner with 1 teaspoon (5g) EVOO.

2 In a small bowl, combine flour, cocoa powder, and baking powder. Set aside.

3 In a medium bowl, using an electric mixer on low speed (or by hand with a large spoon), combine olive oil, applesauce, coconut sugar, eggs, espresso, and vanilla. Add flour mixture a bit at a time, stirring until dry ingredients are absorbed. Stir in ½ cup (240mL) each chocolate pieces and chopped nuts. Gently fold in the raspberries.

4 Spread brownie batter in prepared pan. Sprinkle remaining chocolate and nuts on top of batter.

5 Bake for 25 to 30 minutes, or until toothpick inserted into center comes out with fudgy crumbs.

6 Cool brownies in pan. When cool, lift brownies out of pan onto cutting board. Peel away liner and cut brownies into squares. Store brownies in an airtight container.

PER SERVING: *Calories 165 (From Fat 102); Fat 11g (Saturated 3g); Cholesterol 27mg; Sodium 31mg; Carbohydrate 15g (Dietary Fiber 2g); Protein 3g.*

TIP: Measure all baking ingredients before beginning to save time.

NOTE: I like to double this recipe when making it. I keep a batch in the freezer to serve to guests or to give as hostess gifts.

VARY IT! Swap out the flour for almond flour if desired. If you are allergic to nuts, swap them out for raisins or dried (unsweetened) fruit such as cranberries, cherries, or apricots.

Almond Butter and Cinnamon "Truffles"

PREP TIME: 15 MIN	COOK TIME: 0 MIN	YIELD: 12 SERVINGS

INGREDIENTS

1½ cup (375g) fresh, natural creamy almond butter

2 tablespoons (40g) maple syrup

½ cup (41g) rolled oats

¼ cup (28g) milled/ground flax seeds

1 teaspoon (3g) pure Ceylon cinnamon

1 teaspoon (4g) vanilla extract

⅓ cup (28g) unsweetened dark cocoa

DIRECTIONS

1 In a large mixing bowl add maple syrup, almond butter, oats, flax seeds, cinnamon, and vanilla extract. Mix well to combine with a wooden spoon.

2 Using a spoon or a small melon baller, scoop out the dough to form equal-sized balls. Roll in your hands to make the balls smooth and uniform.

3 Place cocoa on a plate. Roll balls in cocoa and place on a serving platter. Serve immediately or store in the refrigerator for up to a week.

PER SERVING: *Calories 239 (From Fat 180); Fat 20g (Saturated 2g); Cholesterol 0mg; Sodium 5mg; Carbohydrate 13g (Dietary Fiber 3g); Protein 6g.*

TIP: Make these "truffles" in advance and leave them in the refrigerator for up to a week before serving or store in the freezer for up to a month.

NOTE: This decadent dessert provides protein, healthful fats, and carbohydrates so that your blood sugar won't spike after eating them.

VARY IT! You can substitute the cocoa in this recipe for a mixture of ground cinnamon and dried coconut, if desired.

Chocolate Cashew Clusters

PREP TIME: 15 MIN	COOK TIME: 0 PLUS 30 MINS CHILLING MIN	YIELD: 24 SERVINGS

INGREDIENTS

1½ cup (384g) natural, fresh cashew butter

6 ounces (170g) dark chocolate (80% or higher), roughly chopped

10 ounces (284g) cashew, roughly chopped

Fleur de sel, for sprinkling (optional)

DIRECTIONS

1 Set a heatproof bowl over a pan of water over high heat. Bring to a simmer and reduce heat to low.

2 Add the cashew butter and the chocolate and stir until melted and smooth.

3 Add the cashews and stir to coat in the chocolate. Drop 24 rounded spoonfuls onto a waxed paper lined baking sheet.

4 Sprinkle with fleur de sel, if desired. Place the clusters in the refrigerator and chill until firm, about 30 minutes.

PER SERVING: Calories 202 (From Fat 145); Fat 16g (Saturated 4g); Cholesterol 0mg; Sodium 5mg; Carbohydrate 11g (Dietary Fiber 1g); Protein 6g.

TIP: Store the clusters in a covered container in the fridge for up to a week or freeze them for several months. They can even be eaten frozen -right out of the freezer which makes them perfect for serving to last minute guests or whenever you need a healthful treat.

NOTE: These healthful sweet treats make great gifts at holiday time. Both dark chocolate and cashews are diabetes-friendly foods. Peanuts and peanut butter have a low glycemic index, which means they don't cause blood sugar to rise sharply.

VARY IT! Swap out raw blanched almonds and natural, fresh almond butter or peanuts and peanut butter for cashews, if desired.

Pear, Cardamom, and Olive Oil Cake

PREP TIME: 15 MIN	COOK TIME: 45 MIN	YIELD: 10 SERVINGS

INGREDIENTS

⅓ cup (71g) extra virgin olive oil, plus 1 teaspoon (5g) for coating pan

¾ cup (252g) pure agave nectar

3 large eggs

3 cups (336g) almond flour

2 teaspoons (4g) pure ground cardamom

1 teaspoon (4g) vanilla

4 pears, cored, peeled, and diced

DIRECTIONS

1 Preheat oven to 350°F (180°C). Grease a 10-inch (25cm) springform cake pan with 1 teaspoon (5g) olive oil.

2 Place the agave nectar, oil, and eggs in a medium bowl, and mix to combine. Stir in the almond flour, mixing well to combine. Add the cardamom and vanilla, and mix well to combine. Stir in pears.

3 Spoon the batter into the greased cake pan, spread the mixture evenly, and smooth the top. Shake the pan to ensure that there are no gaps in the batter.

4 Bake on the center rack of the oven for 40–45 minutes, or until a knife or toothpick inserted in the center of the cake comes out clean.

5 Remove cake from the oven and allow to cool to room temperature before turning out onto a serving dish. Enjoy at room temperature.

PER SERVING: *Calories 392 (From Fat 234); Fat 26g (Saturated 3g); Cholesterol 63mg; Sodium 22mg; Carbohydrate 36g (Dietary Fiber 6g); Protein 9g.*

TIP: Rustic, farmhouse-style desserts like this one are best enjoyed in the fall, after a meal consisting of a vegetable-based soup and salad.

NOTE: The almond flour in this recipe helps to balance the sweetness.

VARY IT! Use apples instead of pears, if desired.

Oatmeal and Almond Flour Cookies

PREP TIME: 10 MIN	COOK TIME: 10 MIN	YIELD: 22 COOKIES SERVINGS

INGREDIENTS

1 cup (112g) almond flour

½ teaspoon (3g) salt

1 teaspoon (5g) baking powder

¼ teaspoon (1g) pure cinnamon

2 large eggs

1 teaspoon (4g) vanilla extract

¾ cup (162g) Amy Riolo Selections or other good quality extra virgin olive oil

½ cup (100g) sugar

3 cups (243g) old fashioned oats

1 cup (145g) unsweetened raisins

DIRECTIONS

1 Preheat the oven to 375°F (190°C). In a medium bowl whisk together the dry ingredients except the sugar set aside.

2 In a large bowl whisk together the eggs and the vanilla extract. Then whisk in the olive oil until incorporated. Then add the sugar and whisk again until well incorporated.

3 Mix in the dry ingredients and then fold in the oats and the raisins with a wooden spoon or strong rubber spatula. Mix until all ingredients are well combined.

4 Using a small 2 Tablespoon (30mL) ice cream scoop or a 2 Tablespoon (30mL) measure, scoop out the cookies on a parchment lined baking sheet. Then flatten the cookies to about a half inch thick with a rubber spatula. You will likely need to use two baking sheets.

5 Bake the cookies for about 8–10 minutes until the edges are slightly brown and crispy. Remove from the oven and allow to cool before moving them to a cooling rack.

PER SERVING: *Calories 181 (From Fat 100); Fat 11g (Saturated 1g); Cholesterol 19mg; Sodium 83mg; Carbohydrate 18g (Dietary Fiber 2g); Protein 3g.*

TIP: You can prepare the cookies and refrigerate them before baking if needed.

NOTE: If you have nut allergies, swap out oat flour for the almond flour.

VARY IT! You can swap out dark chocolate pieces or unsweetened cranberries for the raisins if desired. Add ¼ cup dark cocoa powder to make chocolate oatmeal cookies.

Chapter **16**

Taking Medications or Supplements

I
f your doctor has just diagnosed you or a loved one with prediabetes, it usually is on the basis of a blood test called HbA1C showing your average blood glucose levels over the previous several weeks. The amount of glucose attached to the red blood cell protein hemoglobin measured in this test show how much excess circulating glucose has been present over a period of time, which in turn reflects levels of insulin resistance — the extent to which the cells in your body have become less responsive to the hormone insulin which efficiently regulates circulating glucose and effectively takes it out of the bloodstream and directs it to cells where it's needed.

An HbA1c level below 42 mmol/mol (6.0 percent) is considered normal, 42–47 mmol/mol (6.0–6.4 percent) indicates prediabetes, and 48 mmol/mol (6.5 percent) or above suggests diabetes. These thresholds can vary slightly between countries and different organizational guidelines.

So, you are possibly wondering what treatment is recommended. This chapter explores the ways to make those changes and when your doctor may suggest intervention with medications or supplements.

Your Prediabetes Management Plan

During the consultation you and your doctor need to agree the best management plan which should have several objectives. These include:

>> Preventing the gradual rise of HbA1c to levels where diabetes is diagnosed

>> Stabilizing, reducing, and normalizing your HbA1c to reduce the risk of complications of prediabetes

>> Assessing and addressing other risk factors for cardiovascular diseases such as high blood pressure, abnormal cholesterol, or chronic kidney disease

>> Arranging regular reviews and follow-up to monitor progress

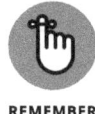

REMEMBER

Although the chances of complications like heart disease, stroke and kidney disease arising from prediabetes are not as high as with the long-term levels of circulating blood glucose seen with diabetes, there is already a small rise in risk of these conditions relative to normal glucose metabolism and an HbA1C below 42 mmol/L or 6.0 percent.

The key to achieving these goals is through reducing insulin resistance. Some factors that contribute to insulin resistance and a rising HbA1C are not possible to alter, such as your genetic makeup or age, but there are several that are modifiable risk factors.

Reducing insulin resistance

Helping your hormone insulin to work more efficiently and effectively by reducing insulin resistance (which is also called *increasing insulin sensitivity*) can be achieved with several key strategies:

>> **Increase physical activity.** Aim for at least 150 minutes of moderate aerobic exercise per week.

>> **Lose excess weight.** Even a 5–10 percent reduction in body weight can improve insulin sensitivity.

>> **Adopt a Mediterranean-style diet.** Rich in vegetables, whole grains, legumes, nuts, healthy fats (especially olive oil), and moderate fish intake.

>> **Limit added sugars and refined carbohydrates.** Reduce sugary drinks, white bread, and processed foods, which is a key component of the Mediterranean diet.

>> **Increase fiber intake — from vegetables, fruits, whole grains, and legumes.** High fiber intake is another central principle of a Mediterranean diet.

>> **Nurture a healthy and diverse gut microbiome.** Encouraged by a Mediterranean diet, your friendly gut microbes increase insulin sensitivity and improve glucose regulation.

>> **Get enough sleep.** Aim for seven to nine hours per night and address sleep disorders such as sleep apnea.

>> **Address stress.** Try to incorporate mindfulness, meditation, yoga, or other stress-reduction practices.

>> **Avoid smoking.** Smoking is associated with higher insulin resistance.

>> **Limit alcohol.** Moderate intake, if any, is recommended. Excess alcohol increases insulin resistance.

>> **Stay hydrated.** Drink adequate water to support metabolism and glucose control.

>> **Avoid prolonged sitting.** Take movement breaks throughout the day.

You and your doctor can discuss how to make these changes and monitor your progress with regular testing of your HbA1C.

Focusing on lifestyle changes

The first line approach to managing prediabetes should always be through lifestyle changes. The benefits go far beyond improving insulin sensitivity and optimizing glucose regulation. They independently reduce the risk of chronic diseases associated with prediabetes and diabetes irrespective of their effects on blood glucose in a variety of ways — reducing chronic inflammation, oxidative stress, improving heart health, and reducing the incidence of many cancers.

TIP

Make sure your doctor has an interest in a lifestyle approach. If your doctor has a special interest or additional qualification in lifestyle medicine, they can support you in achieving these objectives and signpost you to other healthcare professionals if that is appropriate.

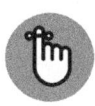

REMEMBER

The objective of your approach to prediabetes is to improve your health and well-being. This approach may be reflected in improvements in measurements or test results such your HbA1C, blood pressure, weight, cholesterol, blood tests for inflammation or resting heart rate. But even if there is little change it doesn't mean that the switches you are making aren't making a difference to your health.

Not everything can be accurately measured through medical tests, but the evidence that these changes have a significant beneficial impact on your health is compelling.

Understanding if medications are recommended

While lifestyle changes such as improving diet, increasing physical activity, achieving a healthy weight or body mass index (BMI), and other factors listed in the previous sections are the cornerstone and most effective approach for preventing the harms and progression of prediabetes, there can be exceptional situations where a doctor may consider prescribing medication.

REMEMBER

In 2025, no drugs are licensed by medicine regulators specifically for use in prediabetes. A doctor can still prescribe a medication at their own discretion. To prescribe a medication "off license" (or "off label") means that the drug is being used for a condition or in a way not officially approved by regulatory authorities, typically because the pharmaceutical company has not sought formal review or licensing for that specific use. When a physician prescribes a medication off license, the responsibility for monitoring and managing any adverse effects falls primarily on the prescribing doctor, rather than the drug manufacturer.

Drugs Sometimes Used for Prediabetes

The decision to prescribe medications is usually based on several factors, including the severity of blood glucose elevation, individual risk of developing Type 2 diabetes, age, weight, history of gestational diabetes, or other health conditions such as high blood pressure, fatty liver disease, or polycystic ovary syndrome (PCOS), and prior unsuccessful attempts to lower blood glucose through lifestyle measures alone.

Metformin remains the most extensively studied and commonly recommended medication for prediabetes. Although officially licensed for the treatment of Type 2 diabetes, it is sometimes used "off label" for people with prediabetes who are at higher risk. Metformin works by enhancing the body's sensitivity to insulin and by decreasing the amount of glucose released by the liver. Clinical trials have shown that metformin can reduce the risk of developing Type 2 diabetes by approximately 30 percent. However, its effectiveness is generally less than that of comprehensive lifestyle interventions, such as those tested in the Diabetes Prevention Program, which achieved risk reductions of up to 58 percent in some groups.

In selected cases, other medications may be considered, such as acarbose, which slows the absorption of carbohydrates in the intestines, or pioglitazone, which improves insulin sensitivity. These drugs are used less often due to concerns about side effects, long-term safety data, and because metformin is usually better tolerated. Newer classes of diabetes medications, such as GLP-1 receptor agonists and SGLT2 inhibitors, are currently being studied for their role in diabetes prevention, but they are not routinely prescribed for prediabetes outside of research or special circumstances. They can however be used for weight loss, which is considered in the next section.

Medication is generally reserved for individuals at particularly high risk of developing Type 2 diabetes such as younger adults with very high BMI, women with a history of gestational diabetes, or those with rapidly rising blood glucose, especially if intensive lifestyle modification does not achieve the intended results. Starting medication involves careful consideration of the benefits and potential drawbacks, such as gastrointestinal side effects with metformin, or bone and fluid retention risks with pioglitazone. It is essential to individualize this choice, balancing the potential to delay diabetes onset against the realities of long-term medication use and the person's own health priorities.

For many people, especially those with mildly raised blood glucose, older adults, or individuals with multiple health concerns, an emphasis on quality of life and avoidance of unnecessary treatment is appropriate. Medication should not replace lifestyle changes, which remain the most effective intervention and have much broader health benefits, but can be a valuable additional tool for those at greatest risk.

Ultimately, the choice to initiate medication for prediabetes should be made collaboratively between the individual and their healthcare provider. Personal preferences, willingness and ability to maintain lifestyle intervention, risk-factor profile, and overall goals of care should all be discussed to arrive at a decision tailored to the person's needs. Regular follow-up is needed to assess progress, side effects, and ongoing motivation for maintaining healthy habits and monitoring blood glucose.

Medicines for other conditions

When you are tested for prediabetes, your doctor should also consider other conditions that may be relevant. Prediabetes and diabetes increase the risk of cardiovascular diseases so you may discuss the possibility of medications being necessary if you have high blood pressure, high cholesterol, or chronic kidney disease diagnosed.

The lifestyle changes we advocate in the chapters on exercise and the Mediterranean diet, which improve insulin resistance, also offer benefits for cardiovascular health including reducing blood pressure and managing cholesterol so medications may not be necessary. However, if your blood pressure or cholesterol levels remain high, or if kidney disease persists, it is possible that your doctor may discuss the need for specific medications for these conditions, especially if your HbA1C remains high.

Weight loss medications

A poor diet and sedentary lifestyle can lead not only to increased insulin resistance and prediabetes, but also weight gain. Excessive weight itself promotes further insulin resistance and so is itself a risk factor for prediabetes and Type 2 diabetes. In Chapter 9, we explore the relationship between a high BMI and prediabetes in greater detail.

In recent years, a new class of medications known as GLP-1 receptor agonists, including semaglutide (brand names Ozempic and Wegovy) and tirzepatide (Mounjaro, Zepbound) have gained widespread attention for their dramatic effects on weight loss. Originally developed and licensed to treat Type 2 diabetes, these drugs work by mimicking hormones that regulate appetite, slow stomach emptying, and improve insulin sensitivity. As a result, they help people eat less and lose substantial amounts of weight, often accompanied by reductions in blood sugar levels and HbA1c. Although not licensed specifically for the treatment of prediabetes, their ability to reduce insulin resistance means they may delay or prevent the progression to Type 2 diabetes, particularly in people with obesity.

Despite their promises, these medications should only be used under close medical supervision, and usually only in people at high risk of developing diabetes who are unable to achieve adequate weight loss through lifestyle change alone. They are not a first-line treatment for prediabetes. Although clinical trials show significant HbA1c reductions and weight loss, there are important considerations. Side effects such as nausea, vomiting, diarrhea, or constipation are common, and there are concerns about longer-term risks that are still being studied. After the medication is stopped, people often regain some or all of the lost weight, especially if lifestyle habits have not changed which raises questions about the sustainability of treatment.

REMEMBER

While these drugs may offer important benefits for selected individuals, the foundation of prediabetes management remains lifestyle change including a healthy diet, regular physical activity, weight loss, and other habits that not only improve blood sugar but also support broader metabolic, cardiovascular and mental health. These medications may have a role for some people, but they should not be a substitute for the long-term advantages of sustainable lifestyle improvements.

Considering supplements

Several dietary supplements are frequently recommended for people with prediabetes, though evidence for their effectiveness varies, and none should replace lifestyle change as the foundation of prevention.

TIP

There's a difference between a doctor recommending a supplement because you have been diagnosed with a deficiency of a particular vitamin or mineral and taking one because of claims that it may help glucose regulation. Having a blood test with your doctor to check levels out is always a good idea.

WARNING

Some supplements may cause toxicity in high doses. It is important that you take advice from a qualified and regulated health professional if you are considering taking a supplement, especially if you have any medical conditions or are taking medications. A lot of unsubstantiated claims are made about supplements so being discerning and seeking guidance if you are in doubt is important. Checking blood tests with your doctor is also important. Home blood testing kits are very variable in their reliability.

The following is a summary of the most commonly discussed supplements and the quality of evidence behind them.

Vitamins and minerals

Vitamins and minerals are essential micronutrients that the human body needs in small amounts to function properly and maintain overall health. Some are involved in the pathways that regulate glucose metabolism and have been studied for possible role in the management of prediabetes.

>> **Vitamin D:** Low levels of vitamin D have been linked with an increased risk of insulin resistance and Type 2 diabetes. Some studies suggest that correcting a deficiency may improve insulin sensitivity, but the results are mixed. Vitamin D supplements, in the form of the most effective "D3 formulation" may be considered if blood levels are low. It is worth getting this checked with your doctor because many people don't get enough outdoor sunshine exposure which is important for vitamin D synthesis.

>> **Magnesium:** Magnesium plays a role in glucose metabolism, and low levels are common in people with insulin resistance. Some observational studies have found that higher magnesium intake is associated with a lower risk of developing diabetes. Supplementation may offer some benefit, particularly in those with a deficiency, though more research is needed. Some medications including drugs called proton pump inhibitors commonly prescribed for indigestion or protection from gastric ulcers can cause low magnesium levels.

>> **Chromium:** This mineral is thought to enhance the action of insulin in the body. Some small studies have shown slight improvements in blood glucose control with chromium picolinate supplements, especially in people with diabetes, but the evidence in prediabetes is limited and inconsistent.

>> **Vitamin B$_{12}$:** While not directly related to prediabetes, vitamin B$_{12}$ deserves mention because long-term use of metformin, a common medication for diabetes and sometimes used for prediabetes, can lead to B$_{12}$ deficiency. Supplementation may be appropriate in people taking metformin or at risk of deficiency (such as older adults or people on vegetarian or vegan diets).

Other supplements

Supplements which are not vitamins or minerals are sometimes promoted for use in prediabetes with claims that they may improve glucose regulation. These supplements are often derived from foods that are thought to improve insulin sensitivity.

TIP

A number of foods have shown to improve insulin sensitivity. These effects are sometimes due to *bioactive compounds* — food components that can positively influence human health, including compounds called *polyphenols*. Bioactive compounds found in whole foods may well be more effective in promoting health than in supplement form due to the "food matrix effect" — the intricate way that various components within a food interact. This influences the absorption, stability, the interface with the gut microbiome and overall activity of the bioactive compounds. The following supplements fall into this category:

>> **Berberine:** A compound found in several plants, berberine has been shown in some small trials to reduce blood sugar and improve insulin sensitivity. It may work similarly to metformin in how it affects glucose metabolism. While promising, berberine can interact with medications and should only be taken under medical supervision.

>> **Cinnamon:** The spice cinnamon has been widely promoted as a natural blood sugar-lowering agent. Some studies suggest it may help reduce fasting blood glucose slightly, but the effects are small and not consistent across all trials. More research is needed before it can be recommended.

>> **Alpha-Lipoic Acid:** This antioxidant may help improve insulin sensitivity. Some studies in people with diabetes show modest benefits. It may also help reduce symptoms of nerve damage (neuropathy) but is not a primary treatment for blood sugar control.

>> **Omega-3 Fatty Acids:** Omega-3s are healthy fats found in oily fish and plant sources such as flaxseed and walnuts. They are known to support heart health, which is important in prediabetes, but most studies have found little or no effect on blood sugar or insulin sensitivity. While not harmful, omega-3 supplements are not currently recommended specifically for preventing or treating prediabetes.

>> **Bergamot:** Bergamot is a citrus fruit rich in antioxidant flavonoids, a type of polyphenol. Some small studies suggest that bergamot extract may help reduce cholesterol and triglycerides and may modestly improve insulin sensitivity. However, research is still limited, and more high-quality trials are needed before bergamot can be confidently recommended for prediabetes.

>> **Olive Oil Polyphenols:** Extra virgin olive oil contains polyphenols, powerful antioxidant and anti-inflammatory bioactive compounds, which may contribute to the protective effects of the Mediterranean diet, linked with a lower risk of developing Type 2 diabetes. Olive polyphenol supplements, such as those from olive leaf extract and concentrated olive polyphenols, have shown modest improvements in insulin sensitivity and inflammation in small studies, but consistent benefits for blood glucose control or diabetes prevention are not yet proven. While promising, they should not replace lifestyle changes and are best considered as part of a healthy diet, especially one rich in extra virgin olive oil.

>> **Probiotics:** The gut microbiome is increasingly linked to metabolism and insulin resistance. Some early research suggests that probiotics may improve blood sugar control by supporting a healthier gut environment.

Chapter **17**

Putting Your Knowledge to Work: A Healthier You in Three Months

I f you read the previous chapters in this book, you know the possible consequences if you let prediabetes progress into diabetes. We give you a lot of advice throughout the book on how to prevent that transition from happening, but what do you do on a daily basis? In this chapter, we integrate the key how-to information in this book into a program that you can follow for three months. This program is perfect for those looking to lose weight, preventing Type 2 diabetes, and improving their health. Discuss it with your healthcare provider to make sure that it is appropriate for you.

Just three short months is all it takes to make significant change in your health. One of the prerequisites for success is that you are emotionally invested in the changes that you are seeking to make. For example, ask yourself the following:

» What's in this for me? How can my life improve if I were healthier?

- What can I enjoy more if I were in better shape?
- What can having good health mean to me?

>> How important is avoiding Type 2 diabetes to me?

>> What can my life look like if I were healthier and in better shape?

REMEMBER

If answering any of those questions is uncomfortable for you or brings up negative emotions, consider speaking to a therapist, counselor, or health coach. Many people have underlying sources of trauma or past experiences that have them feeling stuck and unable to move forward in the direction they'd like. If this is you, speaking to someone can help clear the path to creating the results you desire.

After you have a clear picture in your mind of how you'd like to feel, look, and live, it's time to set the stage. Close your eyes and imagine yourself at your healthiest and best. Let yourself fully experience what it would FEEL like to be healthy and to live out each of the points that you mentioned as answers to the previous questions. What emotions would you experience in the happy, healthy version of you? Imagine how great you'd feel in each of those situations. Repeat this process each morning and night during the three-month program. The more that you can experience the positive emotions of your desired result, the more likely you will be able to achieve your goals.

Try to be in a very positive frame of mind when you start this program. Speaking positively is one matter, and thinking positively is another, especially about yourself. So many people, especially those who are experiencing health problems or weight issues report feeling a tremendous amount of negative emotions including shame and embarrassment. These feelings are harmful and won't provide the inspiration that you need to sustain a healthy lifestyle over the long term. Make a vow to go easy on yourself. Celebrate each small achievement. Every time you do something good for yourself, learn to praise yourself. Whether it's completing a workout, going for a walk, eating a healthier snack, sleeping enough, and so on, each small task is a major win which contributes to a better life for you.

Conversely, if you miss a workout or eat the wrong item, don't be too hard on yourself. Use it as an excuse to accept that you're human and no one is perfect. Affirm the words "Even though I _____ today, I still deeply love and appreciate myself." And then get right back on track when you can. After you know that you're committed, be sure that you have the right environment to begin. Make sure you are ready. If you are not, you won't do well. A week that you're moving, going through surgery or another major life change, for example, is not the best time to begin the program. Do what you can when you can and start when you feel good about it.

After you have successfully followed this three-month program, you will feel much better physically and psychologically. You may want to follow it for an additional three months, or you may be ready for some variety. Either way is fine.

You can make substitutions for the foods we suggest to create a very different diet for yourself. Just make sure you keep the portions about the same so that you end up with about the same number of calories each day.

Getting Ready to Change

Here are a few points you should do to prepare for this program:

» Create your vision of yourself post 3-Month program and commit to it.

» Let your family know what you are doing and ask for their support.

» Download an app that shows your steps taken or use a smart watch, purchase two 5-pound weights, and two 10-pound weights.

» Get rid of the foods in your house that contain the ingredients that make weight control difficult: soft drinks, foods with high fructose corn syrup, and foods with trans fats or hydrogenated oils.

» Commit to avoid eating those same foods outside of the home.

» Stock up on the staples that we list in Chapter 19.

» Have some baseline studies done (see Chapter 9):

- Hemoglobin A1c

- Fasting blood glucose

- Blood pressure

- Cholesterol

- Triglycerides

- Your weight

- Your body mass index

TIP

Discuss with your doctor how frequently you check these measurements to monitor your progress. Do not weigh yourself daily because you may not see much change from day to day. (You'll definitely see change over a two-week period.) Repeat the hemoglobin A1c (HbA1c) at the end of the three months. Record your measurements in a table so you can easily see your progress. Remember that even if your numbers are not changing rapidly, if you are improving your diet and lifestyle, you are definitely improving your health.

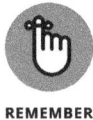

REMEMBER

If you are not perfect on a particular day, don't give up in frustration. Just get back into the program the next day. A few bad days here or there are not going to affect the overall program, especially if most days are good ones.

Following the Plan

You need to learn to walk before you can run. The first month is meant to get you revved up so you can go full speed in month two. Three elements to the change you are making are: the food you are eating, the exercise you are doing, and the behavioral change you are accomplishing.

TIP

During these three months, try to eat at home as much as you can. You succeed much more easily if you do.

Week One

The exercise: Track your steps every day for the first week and just let the steps add up for seven days. Divide by seven to get the number of steps per day. On Wednesday and Saturday mornings, use the five-pound weights to perform the resistance exercises shown in Chapter 17. Repeat each exercise ten times, and then repeat each exercise ten times again.

The meal plan: The diet is very simple and easy to prepare but well-balanced so that you get all the nutrients, vitamins, and minerals you need. The emphasis is on low glycemic foods (see Chapter 12). I provide a sample menu for each week, and you can alter it to provide some variety, exchanging foods of similar nutrient and caloric quality. (We offer suggested substitutions after the sample menu.) For example, instead of ½ cup of apple juice, you can eat an apple or ¾ cups of blueberries or blackberries. Instead of three ounces of skinless chicken, you may eat three ounces of fish or three ounces of veal. Alternatively, so that you know you are following the program exactly, you can do the diet exactly as we have written it every day.

This list is a simple suggestion of ingredient combinations for those looking to lose weight and prevent Type 2 diabetes. Note that the recipes in Chapter 15 are all created to balance blood sugar levels and to prevent the onset of Type 2 diabetes. With adequate physical exercise, they can also help you to lose weight. If you choose to create your own recipes with the ingredients listed in the following plan, here are a few details to keep in mind:

>> **Eat with a friend or loved one whenever you can.** Studies have shown that eating communally boosts mental and physical health. Plan your dining partners just as you would your meals. Even if you're alone, you can make phone or video call meal plans to "eat together" virtually.

>> **For the meats and vegetables, roasting, baking, poaching, and stir-frying in extra virgin olive oil should be your go-to cooking methods.**

>> **Use extra virgin olive oil to add flavor and nutrition to your dishes.**

>> **Dress vegetables with EVOO, fresh lemon juice, a hint of unrefined sea salt, and freshly ground pepper.**

>> **Add flavorful spices to your cooking to boost anti-inflammatory properties:** cinnamon, ginger, black pepper, cumin, turmeric, and chilis are great.

>> **Use lots of fresh herbs when preparing your dishes:** basil, cilantro, parsley, rosemary, sage, thyme, mint, and dill all provide lots of protective bio-active compounds and add taste and depth to your dishes.

>> **Use seasonal fruits and vegetables whenever possible.**

>> **A leafy green salad (or dish of sauteed greens in EVOO and dressed with lemon juice) are a great way to add vitamins and fiber at each meal.**

>> **Use smaller plates and bowls so that your portions, which are undoubtedly less than you are used to, will appear sufficient.** Using blue colored plates is also shown to slow down the appetite and cause you to eat less.

Here is the sample menu:

Breakfast

1 apple

1 piece whole grain toast

1 teaspoon unsweetened almond or peanut butter

1 scrambled or hardboiled egg

1 cup milk

Black coffee, herbal tea, or tea

Lunch

3 ounces skinless chicken

½ cup cooked green beans

4 walnuts

1 slice whole grain bread

1 pear

Dinner

4 ounces fresh fish

1 small baked potato, garnished with EVOO and 4 ounces full-fat Greek yogurt

1 cup cooked broccoli

½ cup cooked beans — black, cannellini, chickpeas, or pinto

⅓ cantaloupe

Salad of green leafy lettuce or spinach or baby kale, tomato, onion, mushroom, celery with 2 Tablespoons extra virgin olive oil and fresh lemon juice as dressing

Snack

¼ cup cottage cheese

½ toasted whole wheat bread

½ cup milk

Following are six substitutions that you can make for each food in this menu to give yourself a variety of tastes for the week

Breakfast

For the apple:

>> ½ banana

>> ¾ cup blueberries or blackberries

>> 12 cherries

>> ½ cup grapefruit juice

>> 2 tablespoons raisins

For the whole grain toast:

>> ½ cup cooked oats

>> ½ cup cooked quinoa

>> ½ whole wheat pita

- ½ whole wheat bagel
- 1 small potato
- 3 tablespoons Grape Nuts

For the egg:

- ¼ cup cottage cheese
- 1 ounce ricotta cheese
- 3 egg whites
- 1 ounce tuna canned in water
- 1 ounce of skinless chicken or turkey

Lunch

For the skinless chicken:

- 3 ounces lean pork
- 3 ounces lean veal (except no veal cutlet)
- 3 ounces wild game, such as venison, rabbit, or squirrel
- 3 ounces pheasant, duck, or goose
- 3 ounces fresh fish
- 3 ounces tuna canned in water
- 3 ounces tofu

For the cooked green beans:

- ½ medium artichoke
- ½ cup cooked or 1 cup raw carrots
- ½ cup cooked cauliflower
- ½ cup cooked eggplant
- ½ cup cooked pea pods
- ½ cup cooked summer squash

For the walnuts:

>> ¼ avocado

>> 12 almonds

>> 2 tablespoons cashews

>> 4 pecans

>> 20 peanuts

>> 2 tablespoons sunflower seeds

The dinner and snack foods can be substituted in the same way: a fruit for a fruit; a vegetable for a vegetable; a meat, fish, or poultry for a meat, fish, or poultry; dairy for dairy; a starch (such as bread) for a starch (such as cereal).

The behavioral change: Give thanks for the food you are eating and envision it healing your body and helping you to look and feel your best while you are eating besides eating: no television, no web surfing, and no reading.

Week Two

The exercise: Do the same exercise as the first week but add 500 steps each day to the average daily steps of the first week. If you averaged 3,500 daily steps in week one, for example, do 4,000 daily. On Wednesday and Saturday mornings, use the 5-pound weights to perform the resistance exercises shown in Chapter 14. Do the resistance exercises for twelve repetitions instead of ten.

The diet: Follow the same program as week one.

The behavioral change: Keep a daily journal listing the food you eat, the exercise you do, and your mood. See Chapter 16 for ideas about how to keep a food record.

At the end of week two, repeat the baseline measurements we describe in the "Getting Ready to Change" section earlier in the chapter (except the hemo-globin A1c).

Week Three

The exercise: Add 1,000 steps to the daily average of week one. On Wednesday and Saturday mornings, use the five-pound weights to perform the resistance exercises shown in Chapter 14. Do the resistance exercises for 15 repetitions instead of 12. In addition, add in a physical activity of your choice that you love once a week. It doesn't matter if it's swimming, water aerobics, dancing, gardening, or golfing. Add in a session a week of whatever you enjoy most.

The diet: Follow the same program as week one.

The behavioral change: Add more water to your diet. Drink water before, during, and after each meal.

Week Four

The exercise: Add 1,500 steps to the daily average of week one. On Wednesday and Saturday mornings, use the five-pound weights to perform the resistance exercises shown in Chapter 14. Add a third set of the resistance exercises so you're doing 15 repetitions of each exercise three times.

The diet: Follow the same program as week one.

The behavioral change: Slow down your eating to make the food last. Put down your fork or spoon between each bite, and don't pick it up until you have swallowed the food. Chew each bite for a long time.

At the end of week four, repeat the baseline measurements we describe in the "Getting Ready to Change" section earlier in the chapter (except the hemoglobin A1c).

Week Five

The exercise: Add 2,000 steps to the daily average of week one. On Wednesday and Saturday mornings, use the five-pound weights to perform the resistance exercises shown in Chapter 14. Do the resistance exercises the same number of times as in week four.

The diet: Follow the same program as week one.

The behavioral change: Find a single place to eat all your food: the designated eating place. It should be a place where you do nothing but eat, such as the dinner table or the kitchen table. Make that space as inviting as possible. Decorate with fun placemats or table linens, use places you enjoy, and add some fresh flowers or a plant to the space to make it more inviting.

Week Six

The exercise: Add 2,500 steps to the daily average of week one. On Wednesday and Saturday mornings, perform the resistance exercises shown in Chapter 14. For the resistance exercises, start using the 10-pound weights but do only two sets of ten repetitions.

The diet: Follow the same program as week one.

The behavioral change: Eat according to a schedule to avoid unplanned eating. Eat three meals a day and a snack daily, or take a little from a meal to have a second snack. If you typically eat alone, be sure to invite friends or family to eat with you a few times this week.

At the end of week six, repeat the baseline measurements we describe in the "Getting Ready to Change" section earlier in the chapter (except the hemoglobin A1c).

Week Seven

The exercise: Add 3,000 steps to the daily average of week one. On Wednesday and Saturday mornings, perform the resistance exercises shown in Chapter 14. Using the 10-pound weights, do two sets of 12 repetitions.

The diet: Follow the same program as week one.

The behavioral change: Challenge yourself to come up with the best flavored versions of the ingredient combinations from the meal plan list. Be sure to load the recipes with fresh herbs and spices. Refer to the recipes in Chapter 15 for suggestions.

Week Eight

The exercise: Add 3,500 steps to the daily average of week one. On Wednesday and Saturday mornings, perform the resistance exercises shown in Chapter 14. Using the 10-pound weights, do two sets of 15 repetitions.

The diet: Follow the same program as week one.

The behavioral change: Keep all food that you are not eating in the kitchen. Don't leave plates of food on counters. Keep leftovers in opaque containers.

At the end of week eight, repeat the baseline measurements we describe in the "Getting Ready to Change" section earlier in the chapter (except the hemoglobin A1c).

Week Nine

The exercise: Add 4,000 steps to the daily average of week one. On Wednesday and Saturday mornings, perform the resistance exercises shown in Chapter 14. Using the 10-pound weights, do three sets of ten repetitions.

The diet: Follow the same program as week one.

The behavioral change: Have snacks pre-portioned in advance so that you can take them with you if needed.

Week Ten

The exercise: Add 4,500 steps to the daily average of week one. On Wednesday and Saturday mornings, perform the resistance exercises shown in Chapter 14. Using the 10-pound weights, do three sets of 12 repetitions.

The diet: Follow the same program as week one.

The behavioral change: Try to choose as much variety in the fresh fruits and vegetables that you consume as possible — aim to "eat the rainbow."

At the end of week 10, repeat the baseline measurements we describe in the "Getting Ready to Change" section earlier in the chapter (except the hemoglobin A1c).

Week Eleven

The exercise: Add 5,000 steps to the daily average of week one. By this point you should be at or very close to 10,000 steps a day. That is the goal. If you are there, you can stay at that level or do more if you want to, but not less.

On Wednesday and Saturday mornings, perform the resistance exercises shown in Chapter 14. Using the 10-pound weights, do three sets of 15 repetitions. You are also at your resistance goal. You can do more repetitions or more sets if you desire, but if you are doing this much, you are accomplishing what you need to.

The diet: Follow the same program as week one.

The behavioral change: When you cook, try making double portions, or more, so that you can have extras on hand for another meal to save time. You may also want to cook in bulk to save time.

Week Twelve

The exercise: You are at or near your goal. Stay at the week eleven level of aerobic and resistance exercises, or do more if you have the need.

The diet: Follow the same program as week one.

The behavioral change: By now you should be avoiding processed and fast food and eating at home as much as possible. If you eat out, keep salad dressing on the side (ask for EVOO and lemon juice instead), limit alcohol to one drink, and avoid bread.

At the end of week twelve, repeat the baseline measurements we describe in the "Getting Ready to Change" section earlier in the chapter, including the hemoglobin A1c.

Applauding Your Accomplishments

If you follow this plan closely, you may accomplish many of the following goals by the end of three months, and it is entirely possible that:

>> You lose between 10 and 15 pounds.

>> You reduce your waistline by one to two inches, most of which is the visceral fat that leads to coronary artery disease.

>> You significantly increase your stamina so that you can perform at a high level for much longer.

>> You significantly increase your strength so that you can easily hoist that carry-on bag into the overhead bin.

>> You greatly improve the quality of your life so that you feel much better about yourself.

>> Your fasting blood glucose can fall by 15 to 25 mg/dL, and your blood glucose after eating can fall by 40 to 60 mg/dL.

>> Your total cholesterol can fall by 20 to 40 mg/dL, and your good cholesterol can rise by 10 to 20 mg/dL.

>> Your hemoglobin A1c falls at least one percent.

>> Your body mass index (BMI) may fall from the obese range into the over-weight range.

>> Your blood pressure falls by 15 to 20 mg systolic and by five to 10 mg diastolic.

>> You feel much more self-assured and able to do whatever you set your mind to.

>> Your thinking is much clearer.

>> You are sleeping much better and feeling much less tired during the day.

>> If you had sleep apnea, you are sleeping soundly.

>> Your joints do not hurt nearly as much.

REMEMBER

Knowledge about prediabetes and diabetes is expanding so fast that great advances are arriving almost daily. Some of these advances may be just what you need. If you can put off developing diabetes for some years, you put off developing the complications as well. You benefit from the *legacy effect,* where control of your blood glucose for several years slows down the development of complications for years after that, even if you later lose your control.

6

The Part of Tens

IN THIS PART. . .

Ten myths about prediabetes

Ten staples to keep in the kitchen

Ten ways to help kids prevent and reverse prediabetes

Chapter **18**

Ten Myths about Prediabetes

Myths about prediabetes and its progression are widespread, creating confusion and sometimes unnecessary fear. Part of the reason so many misconceptions persist is that medical science has evolved rapidly, and old ideas often linger long after new evidence emerges. Public understanding is also shaped by snippets of information from news, social media, and well-meaning but misinformed conversations, which can oversimplify or distort the facts. Health professionals may not be up to date with the most recent developments and sometimes are not particularly interested in the approach of lifestyle medicine which focuses on actionable changes in habits which are often more powerful that the use of drugs or surgery. In this section some of the most common myths are considered and countered.

Having Prediabetes Always Leads to Diabetes

Having the prefix "pre-" in prediabetes suggests that it is a condition that occurs before diabetes and can be interpreted as implying an inevitable progression to diabetes. But this certainly isn't necessarily the case. Studies show that about five to ten percent of people with prediabetes develop diabetes each year. The likelihood of this happening is very dependent on whether any action is taken to reduce the risk factors which are associated with prediabetes and diabetes. Up to 70 percent of people may eventually progress if no action is taken but it's entirely possible to remain stable or even revert to normal blood sugar levels for years with changes in lifestyle habits.

Numerous studies have shown that lifestyle changes such as adopting a healthier diet, increasing physical activity, and losing just five to seven percent of body weight can stop or even reverse the progression to diabetes. Adopting a Mediterranean diet can prevent progression with, or even without weight loss.

Prediabetes Isn't Reversible

With the advice in this book, you can lessen the sugar load in your diet, optimize your body's use of energy for exercise, improve your glucose regulation, and increase insulin sensitivity and the actions of other hormones involved in blood glucose management. The enjoyable lifestyle changes you can make can improve your general health and well-being as well as reduce the risk of prediabetes progressing to diabetes, even if your family history suggests a strong genetic predisposition. Your HbA1C, which reflects average blood glucose levels over time and which currently defines the diagnosis of prediabetes and diabetes, may fall or even fall below the threshold for prediabetes, showing that prediabetes is certainly reversible for some people.

HbA1C Numbers Alone Determine Your Health

Even with an HbA1C in the prediabetes range, you have an associated slight increase in risk of some chronic conditions such as heart disease and stroke. This higher risk of heart disease seen in people with prediabetes is mostly due to other health issues that often occur alongside, such as excess weight with a poor diet, low levels of exercise, high blood pressure, and unhealthy cholesterol levels, rather than high blood glucose on its own. Large studies show that people with prediabetes are more likely to have these common risk factors. When researchers take these factors into account, the direct link between prediabetes and heart problems becomes much weaker, and in some cases, disappears altogether.

REMEMBER

The aim of lifestyle changes is to stabilize and even reduce a raised HbA1C, but even more importantly, it's to improve blood pressure, cholesterol balance, optimize weight and to reduce oxidative stress and chronic inflammation associated with a sedentary lifestyle and poor diet. Doctors don't often measure high sensitivity blood markers of inflammation and oxidized cholesterol, but nevertheless any lifestyle changes will significantly reduce the risk of multiple chronic diseases as well as weight and glucose regulation. Even if you do not bring your measurement into normal range, the changes you are making can definitely benefit your overall health.

A Prediabetes Diagnosis Means that You Can't Enjoy Good Food

A diagnosis of prediabetes is certainly not true that meals become uninteresting or unappetizing. The Mediterranean diet is a pattern of eating that is recommended for prediabetes, with research confirming it's highly effective for glucose regulation, insulin sensitivity, and reducing the risk of developing diabetes. It's also a culinary and cultural heritage that has been shown to reduce the risk of a multitude of chronic diseases including many that are associated with diabetes.

Following the Mediterranean diet is uniquely simple, affordable, pleasurable, delicious, flavorsome, and sustainable. The foods are vibrant and varied with fresh vegetables and seasonal fruit, fragrant herbs, extra virgin olive oil, nuts, seeds, legumes, whole grains, and seafood, prepared in ways that celebrate taste as much as health. Meals are often enjoyed with family or friends, making eating both a source of nourishment and a joyful part of daily life. This combination of enjoyment and proven health benefits makes it one of the easiest long-term strategies for reversing prediabetes and protecting overall well-being.

A Good Diet for Prediabetes Is Just about the Carbs

While the type and amount of carbohydrates you eat does matter for blood sugar control, it's far from the whole story. The quality of your overall diet including the fats, proteins, fiber, vitamins, minerals, and antioxidants such as polyphenols also play a major role in reversing prediabetes and protecting your long-term health. The Mediterranean diet, for example, isn't "low-carb" in the strict sense, yet it consistently outperforms many restrictive diets for improving blood sugar, insulin sensitivity, and heart health. That's because it focuses on nutrient-rich, minimally processed foods including vegetables, fruits, legumes, nuts, whole grains, fish, and extra virgin olive oil, rather than just cutting out bread or pasta. The carbohydrates tend to be low glycemic index and are incorporated in meals with healthy fats and proteins which further lower the rise of blood glucose. It also supports a healthy gut microbiome which is crucial for blood glucose regulation.

TIP

A truly good diet for prediabetes looks at the bigger picture: Nourishing your body, reducing inflammation, supporting a healthy weight, and making food enjoyable enough to stick with for life.

You're at Fault for Your Prediabetes Diagnosis

Many factors beyond personal control can influence prediabetes, and it's not simply the result of "poor choices." Genetics, age, ethnicity, and family medical history can all affect how your body regulates blood glucose as well as other medical conditions or drugs prescribed in certain situations.

Our modern environment also presents challenges. Many jobs require long hours of sitting, ultra-processed foods are widely advertised and easily accessed, and chronic stress can all negatively impact how efficiently insulin works to regulate blood glucose.

The good news is that, regardless of the cause, you have the power to improve the situation. Studies have shown that lifestyle changes such as incorporating more whole foods, exercising regularly, and managing stress, can effectively halt or even reverse prediabetes. The most important matter is to focus on practical steps you can take today, rather than on blame.

A Prediabetes Diagnosis Prevents You from Enjoying Life

This assumption is a misconception. While some dietary plans may feel restrictive, repetitive, and leave you feeling hungry, the approach recommended in this book is different. Combining the Mediterranean diet with appropriate exercise and stress management strategies is not only effective for blood glucose control but also enhances overall well-being including many aspects of mental and physical health.

These changes are not about limitations. They are about improvements and feeling better. Food is celebrated and meals are rich in flavor and variety, physical activity is tailored to be both realistic and fun, and stress management techniques promote a greater sense of serenity and peace. The result is often a boost in mood, increased feelings of energy, and a higher quality of life. Embracing these lifestyle adjustments with prediabetes can lead to a more fulfilling life than before.

Being Thin Is Being Healthy

Social pressure often equates "thin" with "healthy," but the reality about body weight and shape is more nuanced. What really matters is metabolic health, including factors such as blood glucose control, cholesterol levels, blood pressure, muscular strength, bone density, and levels of chronic inflammation, not just the number on the scales. People can be a higher weight and still have excellent metabolic health, just as some people in the "normal" weight range can have poor health markers and an increased risk of diabetes, especially if they have a poor-quality diet.

For older adults, research even suggests that being slightly above the "normal" BMI range can be healthier than being at the lower end, partly because it supports stronger bones, better reserves during illness, and greater physical resilience. The focus should be on building muscle, maintaining mobility, having a high-quality diet such as the Mediterranean diet, and improving blood glucose regulation — not on chasing a thin ideal that may actually undermine your health.

You Can Never Eat Dessert Again

Having a diagnosis of prediabetes doesn't mean you have to give up all sweet treats forever. Whole fruits can be one of the best desserts you can choose, offering natural sweetness alongside fiber, vitamins, minerals, and powerful antioxidants. Because the fiber in fruit slows the release of sugars into the bloodstream, many whole fruits have a low to moderate glycemic impact, making them an enjoyable and tasty choice for people with prediabetes. Pairing fruit with healthy protein or fat-rich foods such as berries with Greek yogurt, apple slices with a small handful of nuts, or fresh orange segments with a square of dark chocolate, can help keep blood glucose levels steadier while still satisfying a sweet craving.

TIP

Some evidence shows that raw, unprocessed honey, when used in small amounts, may offer antioxidant and anti-inflammatory benefits, and it tends to have a slightly lower glycemic impact than refined sugar. That doesn't make it a "free food," but as an occasional natural sweetener in an otherwise balanced diet, especially when combined with foods such as yogurt, nuts, oats, or even a touch of dark chocolate, it can be part of an enjoyable, health-conscious approach.

The key is to focus on desserts that also bring something positive, rich in fiber, protein, healthy fats, or beneficial plant compounds and supportive of a healthy and diverse gut microbiome, rather than ones that deliver sugar and calories alone. With a little creativity, dessert can still be a pleasure, not a problem. For more ideas you can visit the recipe pages in this book in Chapter 15, *Diabetes Meal Planning and Nutrition For Dummies*, *Diabetes Cookbook For Dummies*, and *Diabetes Desserts For Dummies*.

Prediabetes Needs Medication

Currently no medications officially are licensed for treating prediabetes. While some medicines, such as metformin, have been prescribed in very high-risk cases, this is an off-label use rather than standard practice. Lifestyle change remains the first and most effective treatment. Large studies show that healthy eating, regular physical activity, modest weight loss, and good stress management can work better than medications in preventing progression to Type 2 diabetes, while also improving overall health and reducing the risks of many chronic diseases.

WARNING

Some newer weight-loss medications show in research to reduce HbA1C, but their long-term side effects are still being studied. Also concerns that when these drugs are stopped, both weight and blood glucose often return to previous levels. For most people, building sustainable habits around food, movement, and stress management offers safer, longer lasting, and broader benefits than relying on pills.

Chapter **19**

(More Than) Ten Staples to Keep in Your Kitchen

The foods that we feature in this chapter offer a wide array of nutritional benefits, are easy to find, and can be incorporated in various ways into your daily diet. It's a lot easier to eat the foods that are good for you if they are readily available to you. And it's a lot easier to avoid the foods that are bad for you if they are out of sight and out of the house. Plenty of delicious foods keep well in your fridge and pantry. Why not keep them right there where you can prepare a delicious meal without a lot of hassle?

If you need recipes to use these staples, try our book *Diabetes Cookbook For Dummies*, 5th Edition (Wiley). The recipes in that book are not just for people with diabetes but for anyone who wants to eat delicious, healthy food.

Make sure you buy food when they are in season. In-season produce is less expensive and our bodies are actually designed with nutritional needs based upon the seasonality of the produce in the areas that we live.

Extra Virgin Olive Oil

Many studies tout the benefits of eating the *Mediterranean diet* (see Part 4) — the traditional lifestyle followed by people living in the Mediterranean region. Extra virgin olive oil (EVOO) is the common denominator ingredient throughout the Mediterranean and one which is particularly beneficial to those looking to prevent and reverse prediabetes and diabetes.

Extra virgin olive oil (olive oil that has not been refined or industrially treated) is our single favorite ingredient. We actually wrote an entire book on it called *Olive Oil For Dummies* (Wiley 2024).

Olive oil is high in monounsaturated fatty acids as well as polyphenols — compounds which have beneficial anti-inflammatory and antioxidant effect. Extra virgin olive oil, is especially high in these healthy compounds which protect against damage from free radicals and against the formation of cancer. Antioxidants are important in the prevention of aging. Oxidation itself refers to the complex manner in which cells age. Consuming olive oil has been proven to make cells more resistant to oxidation and therefore age more slowly.

Consuming just a few tablespoons a day of EVOO on a regular basis can help prevent diabetes, various types of cancer, heart disease, lower cholesterol, improve rheumatoid arthritis, and reduce the risk of developing Alzheimer's disease. Various studies have shown that regular consumption of extra virgin olive oil can protect against different types of cancer.

TIP

Adding extra virgin olive oil to carbohydrates has the amazing effect of slowing down their absorption in the bloodstream. It also helps to increase insulin sensitivity and helps you to feel fuller sooner. Including extra virgin olive oil in your meals improves gut health and results in a reduced glycemic load. In turn, a lower glycemic load may also play a role in weight management as it can help control appetite and reduce overall calorie intake.

From a culinary standpoint, extra virgin olive oil can be used for drizzling, sautéing, frying, and roasting. You can swap it out for butter or other oils in your favorite recipes.

Green Leafy Vegetables

Leafy greens are an important part of a healthful diet, and you should plan to eat them in as many ways as possible. They can help to fill you up while adding plenty of vitamins, minerals, and antioxidants to your diet. Non-starchy greens such as kale, cabbage, broccoli, cauliflower, collards, Swiss chard, kohlrabi, Brussels sprouts, and dandelion greens are nutritional powerhouses. Try to incorporate at least one serving of them with each meal.

Green leafy vegetables can be sauteed in stir fry, chopped up and added fresh into soups or stews, pureed into soups, roasted with extra virgin olive oil, herbs, and spices, or served in salads. Salad is more than just lettuce and tomatoes. Creative chefs have turned salads into a main course. If you do start with lettuce, choose a dark variety because it contains more nutrients. Here are a variety of greens for your kitchen that provide a variety of nutrients:

» Arugula, also known as *rocket* or *roquette*

» Boston lettuce, also called *butterhead*

» Chicory, which includes *radicchio, escarole,* and *frisée*

» Endive

» Watercress

» Baby spinach or kale

» Dandelion greens

TIP

Store salad greens in the vegetable bin of the refrigerator. Compact lettuce is best stored intact, but loose leaf has to be washed, drained, dried, wrapped in paper towels, and stored in a plastic bag or airtight container to keep it fresh.

You can also store additional prechopped vegetables, hard-boiled eggs, nuts, whole grains, and seeds in your refrigerator so that you can quickly assemble a salad when you need nutritious and delicious fuel fast. Be sure to dress your salads with good-quality extra virgin olive oil and your favorite vinegar or citrus juice instead of bottled and packaged premade dressings which usually contain unhealthful sugars and fats that can derail your eating plan.

Non-Starchy Fruits

One of the biggest misconceptions about eating to balance blood sugar is that you must avoid fruit, and that all fruit is "off limits" and bad for someone with diabetes or prediabetes. This misconception is absolutely not the case. In fact several delicious fruits are included in the "non-starchy" category. They even offer special nutritional benefits for those interested in balancing blood sugar.

A cup of berries packs a lot nutrition and fiber for very few kilocalories (less than 100). You get substances called *bioactive compounds* which include polyphenols such as *flavonoids* that fight cancer. You get other substances that help your vision. The substance that gives blueberries their color, called *anthocyanin*, has been shown to prolong the mental capacity of laboratory animals and may do the same in humans.

TIP

You are much better off getting your berries at the source or at a farmer's market than in the supermarket. In terms of taste, the closer you are to where the berries are grown, the better. If you can find a place where you can pick your own, that's ideal. Otherwise, look for organic varieties. If that isn't an option, or berries are out of season, frozen berries are an excellent choice. They also last a lot longer than fresh berries.

Apples, pears, plums, peaches, apricots, grapes, and other non-starchy fruits are full of fiber, have few kilocalories, and make wonderful desserts. The banana is a starchy fruit, so it is recommended limit yourself to half a banana at a time. That said, everything is relative. We both hear people talk about how bad bananas are for them but yet continue to eat fast food on a regular basis. At the end of the day, any piece of fresh fruit, balanced with a bit of Greek yogurt or almonds for protein and healthful fat, are better choices than processed food.

Tomatoes

When in season, fresh tomatoes are one of the most delicious fruits you can eat. Considered a good food choice for people with diabetes due to their low glycemic index, tomatoes are high fiber content and a rich source of antioxidants, they can be enjoyed by those trying to avoid diabetes as well.

In most areas, tomatoes are in season from July to September. They come in all colors representing all kinds of nutrients, but the main ones are vitamins C, A, and K. You can also get some of your daily potassium needs, as well as some fiber. And the best feature is that despite how good they taste, tomatoes are low in calories.

TIP

The best tomato is one you pick from the tomato plant that you have grown. In warm climates, a few tomato plants can keep an entire family eating tomatoes all summer.

Tomatoes keep beautifully in the refrigerator. They are filled with *antioxidants*, which protect against cancer. Organic tomatoes seem to have more antioxidants than non-organic ones. Eating lots of tomatoes has also been found to lower cholesterol levels.

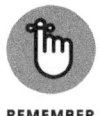

REMEMBER

Drizzling tomatoes, and other fruits and vegetables with extra virgin olive oil increases their nutrient quotient.

Meat, Fish, and Poultry

Unless they are frozen, meat, fish, and poultry do not keep very well. You should buy these items the day of or the day before you plan to eat them. You can also freeze fresh meat, fish, and poultry to have it on hand when you need it.

Fresh fish, especially salmon, mackerel, sardines, and tuna, are fatty fish that are readily available fresh, frozen, or canned. They are excellent sources of complete protein, vitamin D, and other nutrients. The omega-3 fatty acids these types of fish contain along with herring and trout may be specifically important in reducing chronic inflammation. Unless you're a vegetarian, try to incorporate a few servings of fresh fish into your diet per week.

Canned Fish

Canned fish is an excellent way to have fish available at any time. The best are canned salmon and canned tuna fish. Make sure you check the food label for the amount of sodium and for packaging in water. Oil-packed canned fish is very high in calories, and knowing which type of oil was used in packaging is difficult. You can add good quality EVOO to canned tuna which was packed in water. The other thing you want to check the label for is the number of servings per can. Just because the can is small does not mean it is one serving. More often it contains two servings, so you have to share or save the other half for another day.

REMEMBER

Canned fish offers the same health benefits as fresh fish. The oily fishes are protective against heart disease. Canned albacore tuna has the most omega-3 fatty acid, the substance that is protective. When you drain the water, the oil remains in the fish because the oil and the water don't mix. Tuna packed in oil is a different story, however. The oils in the tuna mix with the added oil, and if it is drained, some of the omega-3s are lost.

Canned salmon also provides plenty of omega-3s. Look for boneless, skinless varieties and the more tasty King salmon. Make sure the salmon is wild, not farmed. This way you can have wild salmon all year, not just during the salmon season.

Full-Fat Greek Style Plain Yogurt

Dairy products, including milk, cheese, and yogurt, keep longer than fresh meat, fish, or poultry and are a good source of protein. In the dairy category, full-fat Greek style plain yogurt really stands out in helping to balance blood sugar levels. It's high in protein and vitamin B_{12}, making it a great choice for those who don't eat meat. It contains a significant amount of calcium, B_2, potassium, and magnesium as well. Yogurt with live active cultures (probiotics) is known to help maintain the natural balance of gut organisms. Gut health is particularly important for those looking to prevent or reverse prediabetes or diabetes.

TIP

Try a serving of full-fat Greek style plain yogurt at bedtime to keep you full and your glucose balanced during your hours of fasting. A unique feature of yogurt is that it contains all three macronutrients (protein, fat, carbohydrates) in healthy forms, so you don't have to worry about balancing it out with other ingredients at meal or snack time.

Plain Greek style yogurt can also do wonders in the kitchen. You can swap it out for sour cream in recipes, top with fresh fruit, flax seeds, and nuts for breakfast or a snack, or drizzle some extra virgin olive oil and spices on top for a savory dip to serve with crudites or whole wheat pita bread.

If you can't drink cow's milk because of the lactose, soy milk is a very good substitute. An added bonus: It keeps a lot longer than cow's milk.

Eggs

Eggs had a bad reputation for a long time. Ever since people started checking their cholesterol, they have avoided eggs because each egg contains about 300 mg of cholesterol. But eggs are also a great source of nutrient-rich protein, and they keep very well in the refrigerator.

An egg has only about 75 kilocalories and is packed with nutrients. In addition to the protein, you get choline, folate, iron, and zinc. You can reduce the cholesterol easily by getting rid of one yolk and eating two whites for each yolk.

There are countless ways you can use eggs in your diet. In addition to hard-boiled and poached or scrambled eggs at breakfast, eggs can also be enjoyed in Spanish tortilla, Italian frittata, North African shakshouka, and French-style omelet recipes at brunch, lunch, or dinner.

If you have concerns about egg safety, rest assured that properly cooking eggs makes them very safe. Bacteria are killed as the egg cooks. Make sure no liquid egg is left when your eggs are cooked, and you destroy any bacteria that were hanging around.

Beans and Lentils

Considered the "food of the future" for their small economic footprint, versatility, ease of preparation, and health benefits, beans and lentils are an excellent way to get your protein. In fact, the Mediterranean diet recommends one serving per day of beans or legumes. They are low in fat and high in protein. They contain a lot of fiber, which lowers cholesterol and slows the uptake of carbohydrates. As part of a healthy meal plan, beans and lentils can help you to lose weight and gain muscle.

Dried beans and lentils are available all year and are inexpensive. Before preparing, dried beans have to be soaked in cold water for six to eight hours prior to preparing, so you have to plan ahead. Lentils, on the other hand, only need to be rinsed, but not soaked prior to using. Refer to Chapter 15 for delicious and nutritious ways to prepare beans and legumes.

Both beans and legumes have a neutral flavor which takes on the taste profile of the recipes that they are added to. They can be added to various global recipes such as dips, soups, stews, and salads for enhanced taste and nutrition.

Canned beans, which are precooked, are immediately available for a speedy, delicious meal. But watch out for the extra sodium in canned items. We prefer to prepare the dried variety in large batches to enjoy daily throughout the week.

Nuts and Seeds

From a culinary standpoint, nuts come in a wide variety of tastes and textures. Walnuts, almonds, cashews, pecans, Brazil nuts, hazelnuts, macadamia nuts, and even peanuts (which are considered legumes) are low in carbs and rich in mono and poly-unsaturated fats making them a great snacking option for those looking to balance blood sugar.

The fats in nuts are mostly the good kind: monounsaturated and polyunsaturated fats, which help your heart. From a health standpoint, best nuts include almonds, cashews, pistachios, walnuts, and peanuts. Nuts also contain a lot of vitamin E and fiber. And, of course, nuts keep for a long time.

The U.S. Food and Drug Administration (FDA) has approved a health claim for nuts that states, "Scientific evidence suggests but does not prove that eating 1.5 oz. per day of most nuts as a part of a diet low in saturated fats and cholesterol may reduce the risk of heart disease and cholesterol." The claim is approved for almonds, hazelnuts, pecans, peanuts, some pine nuts, pistachios, and walnuts because these nuts contain less than four grams of saturated fat per 50 grams. Flax seeds, pumpkin seeds, and sunflower seeds also offer these benefits.

While nuts and seeds are a great source of vitamin E, the oil in them starts to turn rancid after they are removed from their shells. If you buy nuts and seeds in their shells, they can last up to a year. Store them in the refrigerator.

TIP

Seeds and nuts are calorie dense, so you have to be moderate in your intake of these foods. You should eat no more than one to two ounces daily, and make sure they are unsalted.

Herbs and Spices

If you're not already packing your recipes with lots of fresh herbs and dried spices, now's the time to start! No better way to add taste to your food (without adding a lot of salt, fat, or sugar) than to add herbs and spices. Plus, herbs and spices contain bio-active compounds called polyphenols which have antioxidant and anti-inflammatory properties that can improve insulin sensitivity and blood sugar control.

Particular herbs and spices, such as cinnamon and basil have been shown to balance blood sugar levels, while others such as ginger, turmeric, and cumin, have efficient anti-inflammatory properties.

Fresh is best, but fresh herbs and spices don't keep long so having a bunch of dried herbs and spices on hand makes great sense. Try them on different foods and see how you change the taste. Here are some that we recommend keeping on hand and using often:

Fresh herbs: You can buy pots of fresh herbs from the supermarket or nursery and keep them on windowsills year round for easy access. Nowadays they even have hydroponic herb growing kits which makes keeping fresh herbs on hand a cinch all year round.

>> Basil

>> Parsley

>> Cilantro

>> Dill

>> Thyme

>> Mint

Dried herbs:

>> Allspice

>> Cayenne pepper

>> Ceylon coriander

>> Green cardamom

>> Cinnamon

>> Cloves

>> Cumin

>> Ginger

>> Nutmeg

>> Oregano

>> Paprika

>> Parsley

>> Red pepper flakes

>> Rosemary

>> Sage

>> Black peppercorns

>> Unrefined sea salt

Chapter **20**

Ten Ways to Stop Prediabetes in Its Tracks

L iving your best life with prediabetes isn't difficult. The more you invest in your health and happiness, the better equipped you are to stop prediabetes in its tracks and prevent it from developing into Type 2 diabetes.

When you realize the power that you hold — through your mind, body, and spirit — to create the life that you want, you can become unstoppable. If you can commit to the possibility of good health, you can look forward to many benefits that you may not have even considered prior to feeling them. With the ten easy steps in this chapter as a guide, you can feel better and prevent further complications down the road.

Adding new tasks into an already busy life is never easy, but if you prioritize feeling good, you'll see that the steps in this chapter offer a high return on your investment of time and effort. We recommend reading through the ten different ideas in this chapter and considering each one with attention and care. Start with the one that seems the easiest for you and begin incorporating it into your life. Say for example, that you love getting outdoors, but may not have "given yourself permission" to spend time outside because of your demanding schedule. Consider this your permission slip! Your health and happiness, coupled with the desire to "stop prediabetes in its tracks," and even reverse it is all the permission that you need to incorporate these items into your daily life.

After you're comfortable with the first idea and you incorporate it into your daily life, pick a second, such as better sleep or maintain a positive attitude. Implement the suggested activities and note how you feel. When they become a habit, move onto the third suggestion, and so on. How quickly you incorporate each item into your schedule is determined by three facets: your commitment to change, your perception of the value of each item in your life, and your personal physical experience. For example, if you are extremely committed to stopping prediabetes from developing into Type 2 diabetes, understand and appreciate that each of the items on this list are essential to making that happen, and have no major physical obstacles (major illness, caregiving, disaster or crisis) preventing you from doing each of these items, you can incorporate them all quickly and see results fast.

If, however, like most people at most times, you have some sort of difficulty which prevents you from sleeping enough or exercising, and so forth, it can take you longer to achieve the desired goals, but you can still see results by taking small steps and doing what you CAN do from where you are. By focusing on the elements you can change, you will feel better and empowered. Little by little, the other obstacles that you have in your life will lessen, and you will be better equipped to deal with those as well.

For each of the suggestions to stopping prediabetes listed here, we offer some modifications and suggestions so that even if they are beyond your reach right now, you may discover ways to slowly implement them. Listing items for people to do in a perfect world is easy, and the truth of the matter is that most adults know eating well, exercising, and sleeping better all contribute to positive health. It isn't because people aren't aware of this that they fail to do them. It's because something gets in the way. Whether the obstacles are perceived ones or physical ones doesn't matter. Anything that causes you to not do what you know is good for you and would like to do is a hurdle that you must be willing to overcome to help yourself enjoy the life you want. This chapter helps you to do that.

Transforming Unhealthy Patterns

So many people are diagnosed with prediabetes nowadays that transforming it should be a part of our everyday conversations. Unfortunately, a social stigma is still attached to people with prediabetes and diabetes diagnosis, and so this topic is avoided. But it shouldn't be. The truth of the matter is that no diagnosis is reason to feel shame. Factors beyond your control have helped to influence the situation of the world and the fact that prediabetes and diabetes have become so prevalent.

So, the first step in transforming unhealthy patterns is to do some soul searching. Ask yourself if you are ashamed of your diagnosis or of the way people may judge you for having prediabetes. If so, do your best to let go of those feelings. "Indulging" in the sense of shame — or any negative emotions for that matter, at this time, will sabotage any healthy lifestyle plan that you decide to embark on. Decide to be kind to yourself as you would be to the person you most care about who came to you and told you that they were diagnosed with something.

The second step in transforming unhealthy patterns should be to forgive yourself for any actions you did to contribute to this situation. If you ate food that you know that you shouldn't have, or not exercised enough, it's okay, we're human and no one is perfect. Accept that our bodies are constantly communicating with us, and a prediabetes diagnosis is your body's warning signal that some issues need to be fixed.

Thirdly, thank your body for taking such good care of you. If you're reading these lines, you can breathe, your heart is pumping, and many miraculous and intricate systems are functioning well in your body, including your vision and your brain, or you wouldn't be able to engage with this book. Thank your body for everything that it provides you with every day, including this internal warning system which is telling you that it would like you to make some changes.

Next, look at the items in this chapter — make a list of which items you are already doing and what you can begin to incorporate next. Start slowly — try to incorporate items one week or every two weeks at a time. Even one new item a month is better than nothing and can still improve your life.

Here are some unhealthy patterns which you can start curbing as soon as possible to prevent prediabetes from turning into Type 2 diabetes:

>> **Believing that you can't become healthy again or that it's too late to change.** This thought simply isn't true — so you can let go of that belief.

>> **Drinking sugary drinks — these are a fast and sure way to spike your blood sugar levels and crave more sugar.** Try giving them up cold turkey — if you can start by replacing one per day with water and continue until you're not drinking them anymore. Replace the "sweetness" that you're giving up in the drinks with other forms of sweetness — spend the time it would have taken you to drink that drink thinking of sweet words that a loved one told you, thinking sweet thoughts about others, or listening to sweet music or lyrics that you love.

>> **Replace fast and processed foods with real foods.** Processed foods are full of sugar, sweeteners, and additives that you don't need and shortens the trip from a prediabetes to Type 2 diabetes diagnosis. If you consume these items

often, vow to replace them, one at a time with real food. Make a list of each time that you eat these items. Has fast food become a quick way to eat a particular meal? Look for quick and easy solutions such as those in this book (see Chapter 15) which give you more value for your money. Is processed food a go to snack for you? Choose a piece of fresh fruit with a handful of almonds or other unsalted nuts, plain Greek yogurt, cottage cheese, hummus and crudites, or a hardboiled egg with vegetables instead.

>> **Figure out what's robbing you of your sleep.** If you're not sleeping enough — look at what you're doing at night before bed. Give up scrolling and late-night TV. Choose instead a relaxing ritual — a bath, meditation, breath work, reading, and so on, which can help you to sleep better.

>> **No time for exercise?** Make a list of everything that you do in a particular day — EVERYTHING. You find times when you're doing activities such as scrolling through social media, watching something on TV, worrying about a problem, and so on. Take back ownership of at least 20 minutes of that time and start moving. Remember that little bits of exertion go a long way to help your body. A few trips up and down stairs or a stroll around the block after meals coupled with parking the car farther away than needed can provide beneficial movement to your body in ways that can add up over time.

We're passionate about helping people transform prediabetes because we believe that through increased understanding, those who suffer from the illness can gain control of their health and situation. Using this book and online resources can empower you to make meaningful choices to improve your health and lifestyle. This book can help you to fully understand prediabetes for the first time, to be less fearful of it, and use knowledge to benefit yourself. The path to optimal health should be a lifelong journey for everyone, not only those suffering from an illness.

WARNING

More information than ever is available due to social media and the Internet. In your quest for knowledge, be sure to seek out solutions from people and resources that are truly beneficial. Remember that a lot of misinformation is available on the web, so you must be careful to check out a recommendation before you start to follow it. Even information on reliable sites may not be right for your problem.

Enjoying the Mediterranean Diet

The Mediterranean diet has been proven to help people prevent diabetes. Those who follow a traditional Mediterranean lifestyle live longer and better — enjoying optimal health late in life. Best of all, the Mediterranean diet is full of delicious ingredients so that you can enjoy a wide variety of foods and feel satisfied while fueling your body with the powerful nutrients it needs to help keep your mind and body sharp and your spirits bright.

If you are what you eat, then you can choose foods that help your body heal and stay balanced. Keep in mind that if you gain weight, you gain insulin resistance, but a small amount of weight loss can reverse the situation. A diabetes-friendly, Mediterranean-style eating plan doesn't have to be a sentence to be excluded from communal meals and gatherings. Actually, communal eating is a tenet of the diet — and eating with others is encouraged.

The same foods that are advisable for someone with prediabetes are also beneficial to anyone seeking to achieve optimal health. Refer to Chapters 14, 15, and 16 to discover all the mouthwatering options that are available to choose from. You can follow the Mediterranean diet from wherever you are, not just at home. Every menu has something on it that's appropriate for you. If you're invited to someone's home, let them know you have diabetes and that the amount of refined and high-glycemic carbohydrates that you can eat is limited. If that fails, limit the amount that you eat.

Here are some details to consider when adopting a Mediterranean diet:

- **Before you decide what or where to eat, decide whom you are going to eat with** — invite co-workers, friends, and family to enjoy your meals with you (no matter how simple they are) as often as possible. If you must eat alone, try talking with someone on the phone or schedule a video call with someone to eat together to enjoy some of the psychological benefits of community.

- **Choose fresh, homemade food over processed and fast food.**

- **Aim to eat six to 12 servings of fresh vegetables and low GI fruit daily.**

- **Drink water as your main drink throughout the day.**

- **Eat three meals a day at set times.**

- **Use good quality extra virgin olive to dress salads, cook with, drizzle on finished dishes such as fish, chicken, meat, and greens.**

- **Choose whole grains — barley, whole wheat, oats, over processed white flour.**

- **Get a serving of beans or legumes per day.**

- **Use fresh herbs, spices, and lemon juice to flavor your food and cook with.**

>> **Use the flavors and traditions of the countries bordering the Mediterranean Sea for inspiration.** You can indulge in Spanish, Provencal, Italian, Moroccan, Lebanese, Turkish, and Greek flavors — just to name a few, so your palate won't get bored!

>> **Enjoy a delicious, homemade dessert or sweet treat once a week as a part of a healthy meal.** Otherwise skim desserts and opt for unsweetened dried fruit such as dates or apricots or fresh fruit or an ounce of dark chocolate when you need a sweet treat.

TIP

A person with prediabetes can prevent it from turning in to Type 2 diabetes with the right diet and exercise. Isn't that benefit worth your effort?

Focusing on Sleep

Sleep has become one of the most undervalued contributors to health in modern society. Many people pride themselves on being so busy (and therefore productive) that they "only have time" for a few hours of sleep a night, as if it were a badge of honor to be sleep deprived.

Other times, we hear about people being sleep deprived because of life crises, illness, or emotional problems. Some people with diabetes may also be diagnosed with sleep apnea or insomnia which compounds the problem, because getting enough sleep is essential to balancing blood sugar.

Getting good quality sleep is essential for maintaining optimal health. While individuals have different needs, for most people getting between seven to nine hours of sleep per night is ideal. Those aged 65 and above should get between seven to eight hours of sleep per night. Inadequate sleep can lead to many health problems including insulin resistance, a condition that disrupts the body's ability to regulate blood glucose and lipid levels. It also decreases the body's ability to burn fat and increases the risk of Type 2 diabetes and increases triglyceride levels.

Here are some tips for improving your sleep schedule:

>> **Go to bed and wake up at the same time each day to regulate the body's internal clock.**

>> **Sleep should not be interrupted so that your body can progress naturally through sleep cycles.**

>> **A cool, dark, and quiet bedroom promotes better sleep.** The ideal temperature is between 60° to 67°F (15° to 20°C).

>> **Limit your exposure to screens and electronics to one hour before bedtime.**

>> **Avoid caffeine and alcohol in the hours leading up to sleep.**

>> **Develop a nighttime ritual** — drinking a soothing herbal tea, writing in a gratitude journal, meditating or praying, taking a warm bath or shower — anything that helps you to relax and feel better.

>> **Choose a light dinner** with foods that are rich in tryptophan, melatonin, magnesium, and omega-3 fatty acids to help you relax. These foods include turkey, eggs, rice, oatmeal, milk, cherries and cherry juice, walnuts, salmon, tuna, sardines, and bananas.

>> **If you need extra help, discuss supplements with a healthcare professional.** Certain supplements such as Magnesium – L-threonate, 5-hydroxytryptophan, melatonin, valerian, chamomile, and lemon balm may have properties which help to promote a better night's sleep. Be sure to check with your doctor, pharmacist, or nutritionist to determine which are best for you and avoid interactions with any other medications or conditions you may have.

>> **Have your hormone levels checked and seek the proper care to balance them if needed.**

>> **Regular exercise promotes better sleep by reducing stress and anxiety.**

>> **Consider taking naps.** In addition to a good night's sleep regular naps are very beneficial to health. They can help you to increase alertness and productivity, improve overall sleep time, avoid afternoon slumps, and balance your hormones. Ideal nap times are believed to be ten to 20 minutes. Drinking a cup of coffee or tea before a nap can help you to not nap for more than 30 minutes so that it won't interact with your evening's sleep.

Getting Enjoyable Exercise

Exercise is an easy, effective, and free way to stop prediabetes in its tracks. Many people have reversed prediabetes and Type 2 diabetes with a healthy diet and lifestyle. Others have had Type 2 diabetes for decades and have little trouble balancing their food and insulin. They're the enthusiastic exercisers. They use exercise to burn glucose in place of insulin. The result is a much narrower range of blood glucose levels than is true of the insulin takers who don't exercise. They also have more leeway in their diet because the exercise makes up for slight excesses.

It doesn't take an hour of running each day or 50 miles on the bike to be healthy. Moderate exercise, such as brisk walking, can accomplish the same goal. The key is to exercise faithfully. (For more on exercise, see Chapter 10.) Thirty minutes of moderate exercise every day not only improves your diabetes but also reduces the possibility of a stroke, a heart attack, and many cancers and just keeps you feeling generally good. Exercise can reduce your hemoglobin A1c (HbA1c) by one percent or more, just like diet can.

TIP

Before embarking on a new exercise plan, discuss it with your doctor to make sure that it is safe for you.

An hour a day of moderate aerobic exercise (something you can do without getting out of breath) provides enormous physical, mental, and emotional benefits. It can cancel the negative effects of reduced activity and eating. Be sure to warm up and cool down for about five minutes before and after you exercise.

You may be getting exercise and not be aware of it because it's not done in a gym! By picking forms of exercise that you love you can reap even more benefits. Walking, running, playing team sports, swimming, skiing, tennis, aerobics, dancing, and golfing are all good forms of exercising.

For best results, vary the types of exercise that you get, aim to exercise daily. Exercising outdoors offers even more benefits, as does exercising with others which adds the benefits of community to your routine.

Spending Time Outdoors

According to one government estimate, Americans spend more than 90 percent of their lifetimes indoors. Outdoor time, however, can improve overall health and mental wellness. Increased digestion, better immunity, improved mood, and reduced risk of illness are all benefits of spending more time outside. If you want to stop prediabetes, or any other illness in its tracks, engaging with nature more often is a good idea.

Natural light helps people to heal faster. Hospital studies have shown that patients with a view of trees outside their windows recovered better than those staring at a brick wall, and when fresh air was added to the mix, the results improved even more. Light also elevates people's moods, so being outdoors can lead to more positive emotions. Just five minutes of exercise in green spaces can improve both self-esteem and mood.

Mental health experts recommend 30 minutes of fresh air a day — and many believe that it's more beneficial to the psyche than antipsychotic drugs. Because maintaining a positive attitude, which we discuss in the next section, is a key player in reversing diabetes and preventing prediabetes from turning into a Type 2 diagnosis, fresh air should be one of your top priorities.

Some ways to increase outdoor exposure include:

>> Finding an outdoor activity that you love and "giving yourself permission" to do it — whether it's planting a garden, golfing in the summer or skiing in the winter, going for a walk with a friend, or just sitting outside and enjoying a meal with others, you will be healthier for it.

>> Give your indoor time "outdoor" access by spending time close to windows and with windows open.

>> If there are parks in your area, go for a quick walk, or sit outside to read, check social media, or enjoy a picnic.

>> Take anything you can do outdoors, outdoors; writing, eating, talking, phone calls, and so on, all give you increased outdoor time.

Maintaining a Positive Attitude

Your approach to life can go a long way toward determining how well you live with your diagnosis. Adopting the mentality that you can stop prediabetes in your tracks is important and that you are capable and worthy of healing. If you have a positive attitude and treat the prediabetes diagnosis as a challenge and an opportunity, stopping it in its tracks will be easier for you.

With the right mind set, your body can actually produce chemicals that make healing happen. A negative attitude, on the other hand, results in the kind of pessimism that leads to failure to diet, failure to exercise, and failure to take your medications. Plus, your body makes chemicals that are bad for you when you're depressed.

Prediabetes is a challenge; to prevent it from turning into Type 2 diabetes, you may have to think about doing certain tasks that others never have to worry about. Eliminating processed foods, finding time to exercise, enjoying healthful meals, and focusing on yourself may be actions that you've never done before. If so, don't worry, you aren't alone. Many of the healthiest, happiest, and most fit people got that way after "wake up calls" with their health.

Remembering that the human body constantly provides feedback is important. When you feel your best, it's telling you that you're doing the right things, and the way you feel is your proof. When you don't feel your best and are experiencing mental or physical discomfort of any kind, your body is signaling you that it needs something to be different. Instead of catastrophizing that the diagnosis is something bad, look at it as an opportunity to make things right with your body.

How would you like to feel? Do you believe that the suggestions in this chapter (and book) can help you to transform a prediabetes diagnosis into optimal health? If you can first accept that truth, and then incorporate the steps outlined, you can feel better than before your diagnosis, perhaps better than you ever did before, and you will set yourself up with a lifestyle that can have you living your best life.

The roadmap to optimal health is not overnight, but the good news is that the sooner you start out on your journey, the sooner you will see and feel results. The need to improve your health may help you tap into your organizational skills, which can then be transferred to other parts of your life. When you're organized, you accomplish much more in less time. A prediabetes diagnosis offers you opportunities to make healthy choices for your diet as well as your exercise. You may end up a lot healthier than your neighbor who doesn't have prediabetes.

TIP

Feeling gratitude is the fastest way to improve your state of mind. Whenever you are upset about something, take deep breaths. Make a conscious decision to put that (or those) issues aside or hand them over to a higher power. Turn your attention to the things that you are most grateful for. Spend a few minutes focusing on each one. Imagine your life without it, and the reasons why you are grateful for it. Repeat each time you need to shift emotional gears from negative to positive.

Celebrating Your Community

A strong sense of community is one of the keys to success of the people who live in areas known for health and longevity. Our communities can give us a stronger sense of belonging, safety, and pride when fully embraced. Nowadays, especially in the United States, our sense of community has diminished. Many people feel more connected to online groups and social media accounts than they do to actual people. If that is true for you, then it may take a bit of effort to embrace a physical community.

Community can be centered around the place you live, work, worship, or with people with whom you share a common interest such as a sport or art form. Community can be made up of family members, friends, or those who share similar interests. And yes, even though it shouldn't be an exclusive replacement for physical community, online communities can also add support to our lives.

Did you know that eating communally is at the foundation of the Mediterranean diet — named the healthiest diet in the world — because it is shown to improve mental and physical health? Exercising communally, attending social events, and developing friendships with those who live in the same area or frequent the same places can be deeply rewarding and help to improve your health.

If you are looking to build a community to enjoy, here are some tips:

>> Determine whether you have enough friends or family in your area that you can engage with more often.

>> Do you have co-workers with similar interests that you can attend social events with or take walks or exercise with?

>> What are your interests? In many areas you find meet up groups focused around shared interests such as languages, the arts, sports, and so on.

>> Does your place of worship or residence offer social outings or group activities that you enjoy?

>> Are you involved in any online groups with similar interests? Whether you're a fan of history, archeology, music, there are Facebook and Instagram groups that offer fuel for your passions.

By becoming part of these groups, you can increase your socialization with like-minded people. Over time, you will have created your own community, based on familial or friendship bonds, or even similar interests. These relationships can go a long way to support your mental and physical health.

Developing Ways to Cope with Stress

Stress can't be avoided. Because the more you focus on something, the more it grows, accepting that stress is a part of life is best. It's our response to stress that can improve our health and stop illnesses and diagnosis such as prediabetes from worsening. Take a minute to think, truthfully (this is just for your own information) about how you currently cope with stress. When you get bad news, feel overwhelmed, or have a new obstacle thrown at you, what is your first response? If you become frustrated or worried, you are like most people.

Think about the first action you take; do you reach for a sweet treat, drink, or treat? Do you eat junk or fast food? Do you stop everything and freak out? Maybe you lay down in defeat or immediately call or text someone to share "you won't believe what just happened to me!" Each of these responses is normal and valid and shows you what you need in that moment. Try keeping a notebook with you and logging down what you do when you are stressed. At the end of a week's time, you may be surprised to read your entries, and whatever you wrote holds the keys to transforming your coping mechanisms.

For example, if you immediately reach for something sweet to eat or drink, you will be able to see that your blood sugar levels are tied to a stress response. You can make a conscious effort to replace the unhealthy sweetness with safer alternatives. This adjustment can look like a combination of things. Once a day, allow yourself a "healthful" sweet treat as a coping mechanism such as a piece of ripe or unsweetened dried fruit, or honey topped plain Greek yogurt. Another time, instead of opting for food or drink, try listening to a sweet song, a beautiful poem, or reminiscing on the sweet words that a loved one told you, or that you would like to hear. Use "sweet" positive affirmations for yourself.

If you turn to junk and fast food in times of stress, think about the reasons why. Are these foods somehow seen as "rewards" in times of stress? Do you associate happiness or good memories with them? If so, make yourself a list of healthy things that have real rewards attached to them, such as the items on this list, and opt to do them instead.

Do you tend to call someone to complain when stressed? Instead, try writing or typing what is making you the most upset. Get it down on paper, read it aloud and notice how it bothers you. Then tear up the page and say to yourself, aloud, "this is over." Throw the paper away, get a glass of water, and write down the opposite. Write the same story in the way that you'd like it to be, in present tense, as if your desired outcome were true. Imagine that it were happening. Now call your friend. Talk about your dreams with them, what you'd love to have happen, or another (positive) subject entirely.

This isn't to say that you can't call friends and ask for help and support. There are times for that too. If you have supportive, and trustworthy friends, you should call them and ask for support when you need it. The activity described above is simply to break the habit of calling to complain, which often leads to more complaining, and a negative frame of mind.

Here are some healthy ways to cope with stress:

>> Look for more things to laugh at — watch comedies, joke with friends, try to look for the funny aspects of life.

>> Exercise daily — for all the benefits mentioned previously and because it helps you cope with stress.

>> Develop a list of healthy activities that you can do when stressed to feel better and refer to it as needed.

>> If it is a major stressor, seek support from a therapist, health coach, confidant, and loved one (perhaps all) to help support you through the difficult time.

>> Try to get enough sleep.

>> Mediate and do breathe work.

>> Practice gratitude, prayer, and/or positive imagery which are all shown to help reduce stress.

>> Eat balanced meals.

Embracing Meal Planning

To prevent prediabetes from turning into Type 2 diabetes, it's important to plan your meals — no matter where you eat them. Be sure that you aren't going more than five waking hours without a nutritious, balanced meal or snack. Each of those should include lean protein, healthful fats, and quality complex carbohydrates to prevent your blood sugar from spiking.

Your meals should include extra virgin olive oil, fresh fruits and vegetables, and lots of fresh herbs and spices for their bioactive and healing properties. Choose from the plant-based foods (fruits, vegetables, beans, legumes, seeds, nuts), lean poultry, meat, and fish to make up the majority of your meals.

Planning meals doesn't just involve deciding what to eat, it requires finding the adequate time for shopping for food, prepping ingredients, cooking, storing food, and planning ahead. Take a look at your schedule and determine when you can do each on a weekly basis. If you're not used to making food at home, it may be a challenge at first, but one that is well worth the effort.

Having a plan to deal with the unexpected is so important. For example, say that you're invited to someone's home, and they serve something that you know will raise your blood glucose significantly. What do you do? Or perhaps you go out to eat and are given a menu of incredible choices, many of which are just not for you. How do you handle that? Or when you run into great stress at work or at home, do you allow it to throw off your diet, exercise, and compliance with your doctor's orders?

A little advance planning can overcome any eating challenge. Discuss good foods with the people who regularly cook and eat with you. Check out Chapters 8, 12, 14, and 15 for more information. You may want to consider reading *Diabetes Meal Planning and Nutrition For Dummies*. Make a meal plan that works for you and follow it.

TIP

The key to a good meal plan is realizing that not everything goes right all the time. In the case of the friend who cooked the wrong food for you, you can eat a small portion to limit the damage. At the restaurant, you should come prepared to make the food choices you know can keep you on your diet. It may be better not to look at the menu and simply discuss with your waiter what is available from your list of correct foods. With these strategies in mind, you'll be prepared to make choices while dining out that will help to keep your blood glucose levels balanced.

Cooking Delicious and Nutritious Foods at Home

The people who make healthful meals at home always have an advantage over those who purchase them (even if they are labelled "healthy") from outside. Cooking your own foods enables you to control what the ingredients you use. Not only can you ensure that you're not loading them with ingredients that can raise your blood sugar and inflammation, but you can also choose to include ingredients known to balance blood sugar and decrease inflammation — such as those in Chapter 15.

If you're not a fan of cooking already, our best advice is to find the best way to embrace it. A lifelong love affair with healthy food can safeguard your health. If you're someone who likes challenges, then accept that cooking is good for you, and challenge yourself to come up with the tastiest versions of nutritious food possible. As a young girl, Chef Amy decided that because she had to cook, she may as well enjoy it. She challenged herself to do the best with the ingredients her mother gave her, and it led to her career. You probably have no desire to be a professional cook, but stopping the progression from prediabetes to Type 2 diabetes and other health complications and being able to enjoy food that is both good for you and delicious (which is hard to do when eating out) should be inspiration enough to get you to spend more time in the kitchen.

Chapter 15 is full of recipes for all palates, seasons, and occasions that you can use as templates to create your own specialties and family favorites. In modern society, time is seen as the number one obstacle to home cooking, but the truth of the matter is that there are 168 hours in a week. If you spend 56 sleeping and 40 working, there are 72 hours left over. If you spend one of those hours meal planning, two of those hours shopping for food, one of them meal prepping, and seven (one hour per day which is more than needed) cooking, you still have 61 hours left over. Add in an hour a day of exercise, and you still have 54 hours.

The truth of the matter is that there are very few pursuits that you can spend time on which can have a better return on investment than preparing nourishing and balanced meals and exercise. Commit to those activities and guard the "quality time" associated with doing them as if your life, health, and happiness depended on it, because it does.

TIPS TO MAKING POSITIVE CHANGES EASILY AND EFFECTIVELY

Here are some tips to keep in mind when incorporating each of these items:

- Commit to wanting to implement these items to prevent prediabetes from turning into Type 2 diabetes.

- Carefully read through each of these items and take notes — are there steps that you're already taking? Are there any items which you have an aversion or a physical or psychological limitation which prevents you from doing them? Any practices that really look exciting to you?

- If there's anything you're already doing — congrats! You're one step closer to your goals. Pat yourself on the back and write it on the list of positive actions that you are going to incorporate into your daily life from now on.

- If there's anything you have an aversion to — for example, you don't like exercising, you don't want to change your diet or prepare food at home, consider the benefits of each one of them. Is it worth doing something that you don't love to enjoy optimal health? Is there a way you can make those items more likeable? For example, if you hate to exercise in general, would you find walking outdoors or dancing or gardening pleasurable? If so, adopt those items first. Do you despise preparing food at home? Is that amount of discomfort greater than the symptoms that you feel if you develop Type 2 diabetes? Probably not.

- If the thought of implementing one of the items on this list is so difficult that you feel you can't overcome it on your own, seek the help of a therapist, health coach,

(continued)

(continued)

physical trainer, or psychologist who can help you overcome it. This solution may seem extreme, but often psychological patterns prevent people from achieving their goals. Sometimes this one step alone can be the key to success when it comes to making positive changes. By investing the time to get to their root causes, you free yourself from being a victim of them and being doomed to a life of physical discomfort.

- Do you have physical limitations to any of the items on this list? In each section we offer suggestions to common obstacles, but in the worst-case scenario, if there is truly something that you can't do, just begin with what you can.

- Make a list of each of the items that you plan to do daily and read it each morning to yourself.

- At the end of each day, in your gratitude journal, make a list of the items that you did to positively impact your health and congratulate yourself for each — no matter how easy they are.

- Reward yourself continuously. Speak kindly to yourself and tell yourself "I'm proud of you for _____" and "I'm grateful that I was able to ____ today." Repeat affirmations such as "I'm happy, healthy, and free" and "I love and approve of myself" as often as possible. By saying these positive affirmations, you set the tone and the pace for the way that your mind and body respond to you.

- Give thanks for everything you can as often as you can. Gratitude is a powerful magnet which attracts goodness into our lives.

IN THIS CHAPTER

» **Making good food that appeals to children**

» **Enjoying cooking and baking**

» **Getting enough exercise**

» **Taking time to rest**

» **Spending time outdoors and with family**

Chapter **21**

Ten Ways to Help Kids Prevent and Reverse Prediabetes

Technically speaking, preventing and reversing prediabetes in children isn't much different than doing so in adults. What's different, of course, is that children think differently and don't have the fully developed reasoning capacities that adults do. It's harder to make a children appreciate why eating well, exercising, and spending time in nature or with others will benefit them in later years. To their benefit, however, kids haven't been alive long enough to practice unhealthy habits as long as some adults have.

Children are also highly impressionable, meaning that they model themselves after adult behavior. Regardless of whether your own lifestyle is healthy or not, your children want to emulate what you do. For this reason, it's important for you to "buy in" to whatever strategies you're trying to get your kids to do before trying to convince them to do so. You can tell children to choose an apple over chips over and over again, but if they see you eating chips on a regular basis and never enjoying an apple, it will be hard to convince them. Alternately, if a child sees their parents or caregivers consistently enjoying healthful foods, they will want to do the same.

Before "putting your kid on a diet" or restricting what they do, examine your own eating patterns. As you read through the suggestions in this chapter, think about whether you can make these changes on your own. If you adopt them and appreciate the good that they can bring, you can be much more successful in getting your children to follow them as well. One successful example is to embark on new lifestyle habits as "an adventure." Turn the following tips into ways in which you can bond with your children. Kids crave attention much more than they crave any type of processed food. If you can give them more shared experiences in general, you will set them up to make healthier choices in other areas of their life.

Exercising, socializing, cooking, baking, playing sports, dancing, singing, playing games, and getting outdoors together are the best ways to show your child that you support them.

REMEMBER

Promoting a healthy weight in children is crucial for preventing conditions such as prediabetes. But approaching this positively is equally vital by emphasizing balanced nutrition and active lifestyles without inadvertently fostering anxieties that can lead to eating disorders.

Revolutionizing Real Food

Using diet, exercise, and other lifestyle hacks, prediabetes can be reversed. A great place to start is to revolutionize the way that you eat. Because we know that processed foods packed with sugar, sodium, and fat can contribute to the onset of diabetes, a first step is to eliminate them from your diet and from the diet of your children. If you are used to eating a lot of processed and fast food and sugary drinks, this may be difficult at first. You (and your child) may crave the ingredients and additives that your body's become accustomed to from consuming these foods. If this is the case, it can be especially beneficial to add vibrantly colored fresh fruits and vegetables, citrus, fresh fish, and polyphenol and antioxidant-rich extra virgin olive oil, spices, and fresh herbs into your diet. See Chapters 8, 12, 13, 14, and 15 for more information and ideas on specific beneficial ingredients, dietary suggestions, and recipes.

Another challenge is the convenience factor. If you're not used to cooking or preparing fresh food, you have a learning hurdle that is worth it. In our lectures and workshops, we like to help people prioritize eating well. The processed food industry has trained generations of people around the globe that "convenience" food is favorable to other options. This habit is not the case. Saving 15 or 30 minutes a day in the kitchen is not the better choice when it costs you your health by leading to blood glucose spikes, higher cholesterol, mood swings, heart disease, and much more. We could write a book on this topic alone, but you get the picture.

To reverse prediabetes and prevent yourself and your children from developing full blown diabetes and other health risks, you must become revolutionary in the way that you treat nourishment. Just like any historical revolution, joining the real food movement requires the adaptation of a new mindset. Don't settle for large companies and the mass food industry telling you and your family what they need and when. Stand up for your health and the health of those you love. Prioritize your children's nutrition knowing that what you feed them can either make them sick or make them healthy. After you realize that every morsel of food that goes into their bodies can help or harm your children, you will be inspired to make healthy choices for your children.

In our careers as a doctor and a chef, we have witnessed many children make the switch to healthful eating for themselves. Kids like to be treated as adults. By teaching kids the truth about nutrition with a convinced mindset, they will appreciate your care and concern. Sure, kids have pressure to do "what the other kids are doing," but the key is to make them aware of other kids who are doing things the right way. At one point in her career, Chef Amy "adopted" a 3rd grade class in an elementary school in Washington, DC. As "their chef" she was asked to help the kids cook and enjoy the vegetables that they harvested in their gardens.

On the date of her first cooking demo, she learned that kale and collard greens were the only vegetables available to her. She feared that the kids would boo her off the stage. In anticipation of the class, she thought about her own life and the best kale and collards she ever tasted. She thought of an Ethiopian recipe which included the greens sauteed in lots of onions, garlic, chilies, red pepper, and ginger. She decided to prepare that recipe for the class. To get them excited about the recipe, she prepared a PowerPoint presentation about farm kids in Ethiopia who also ate greens. Then she made the recipe, which was highly nutritious, but definitely not "normal" American kid fare. Sensing her enthusiasm for the recipe, the 3rd graders were very engaged in the process and ended up loving the dish. In fact, they liked it so much that they asked for seconds and asked for leftovers to take home to their parents "who had never eaten greens before."

While this example may seem a bit dramatic, it exemplifies the need to get passionate about healthy eating perfectly. By spending a bit of time in the beginning by thinking of how to make the kids like the recipe at hand paid off by "selling them" on something very healthful. Look at it this way, the multi-million-dollar advertising campaigns (which are created to convince us to consume foods that are not good for us) invest a lot of time into making these ads. Why not invest some time in creating your own "campaigns" to revolutionize the way we eat and take charge of our health?

Good for You Alternatives to Unhealthy Favorites

Now that you joined the "real food revolution," it's time to develop some quick swap outs that you can have on hand to offer kids. Note that there is a lot of psychology involved in determining what we want to eat. When you couple the psychology with cultural norms and expensive advertising by fast food companies, it's no wonder kids seem to gravitate toward unhealthy foods.

We see experts advise kids to avoid junk food until their prediabetes diagnosis is reversed. But it is much better for them to steer clear of junk food on a regular basis forever, in order to avoid another diagnosis down the road. The goal isn't to get healthy in the short term, it's to learn to eat foods that do the body the most good to look and feel your best. Speaking to children honestly and directly about the healing properties of food and the importance of diet (See Chapters 2, 4, 8, 12, and 13) gives them the tools they need to live and eat with both pleasure and health in mind.

One taste profile that everyone craves is sweetness. This craving is because mother's milk is sweet, so we, as humans, literally learn that the sweet taste is associated with comfort, safety, and nutrition as infants. Sweet flavors continue to remind us of this our whole lives and we continue to crave them. One trick to satisfy our sweet tooth and to enjoy nutritious foods is to incorporate foods that are naturally sweet, and to balance them with healthful fat, lean protein, and so on.

Sugary treats aren't the only way to add sweetness into our lives. Speaking to your children with positive, kind words, by teaching them to practice gratitude and to engage in feelings they love can help to curb the emotion-based triggers for sweets and comforting carbohydrates.

Here are some swap outs to make healthy eating more enjoyable for kids and adults alike (see Chapters 4 and 8 for more details):

>> Extra virgin olive oil (EVOO) for butter

>> Greek yogurt for sour cream

>> One serving of fresh fruit instead of fruit juice

>> Water instead of soda or sweetened drinks

TIP

Children must learn how vital water is to their health. Avoid starting your child on soft drinks at all costs. Encourage them to drink water before, during, and after each meal. Sugary drinks (even if they're made with sugar substitutes) aren't just devoid of nutrients, they are harmful to kids. By eliminating them from your child's diet, you are doing them a favor. Children should appreciate that the best thirst quencher is water. Make sure your child has easy access to water all day long.

>> Unsalted roasted nuts instead of chips

>> Oatmeal and whole grain instead of boxed cereals

>> EVOO, vinegar, and lemon juice instead of bottled salad dressings

>> Homemade desserts versus store bought on occasion

>> Protein rich snacks such as Greek yogurt, ricotta cheese, edamame, and bean-based dips versus empty calories

>> Swap out dark chocolate — 80 percent or higher — for milk chocolate

>> Swap out natural sweeteners — raw honey, pure maple syrup, and date sugar instead of table sugar (and use them sparingly).

>> Homemade versus store bought

TIP

Remember, just a few healthy swaps alone can go a long way to helping your kids. If people know which foods are better options but still prefer unhealthy food, it's worth investigating the psychological feelings behind their choices. If parents are doing everything in their power to get kids to follow a healthy eating plan (including following and enjoying one themselves) yet the kids won't budge, seeking out counseling is worthwhile.

Hero Foods

Kids look up to heroes — whether they are action figures, sports stars, athletes, or celebrities, many of these public figures pay attention to diet and exercise. Kids need to learn from a young age that it is the bioactive compounds in fresh produce that give them the nutrients that they need to supercharge their own diets and have them feeling supercharged.

Choose to empower their dietary choices by keeping fresh vegetables on hand and preparing them in as many tasty ways as possible. Per the Mediterranean diet (see Chapters 12 and 13), we should all be eating 9-12 servings of fresh produce per day. In fact, these are the ingredients that our diets should be based around — with healthful sources of protein and fat added in.

Get kids involved in the choosing and cooking process whenever possible. Take them to farm stands, farmer's markets, and even farms to learn how crops are grown, or show them specials on TV. Teach them how good these vegetables are for you and how you can prepare them to make them taste great, because if you don't, this is not information that they will learn elsewhere. Commercials and social media campaigns aren't built around vegetables, they're focused on mass-produced ingredients in boxes or that can be purchased at a fast-food restaurant, so kids usually crave those.

Celebrating local fare

In Italy and in other places in the Mediterranean, large community-based festivals are held in honor of different types of produce that are important to the area's economy. Everything from chili peppers to artichokes and chestnuts have festivals in their honor. These *sagre* as they are called date back to pagan times when agrarian gods were praised for providing ample crops. Nowadays some of them have gotten so popular that they attract tourists from around Italy and the world and include musical bands, hundreds of stands selling different dishes based on the food being celebrated, games for children, dancing, folkloric traditions, and more. These traditions help to pass down the love for seasonal produce on to children. In the areas where these festivals are held, most kids have a good idea of many ways to enjoy each type of produce by the time they're eight-years-old — and they don't need to be forced to do so.

In other places of the world, it's not so easy. But if parents and caregivers really become convinced that produce is the way to go, they can make eating fresh fruits and vegetables just as interesting for kids anywhere as those in the Mediterranean region. If this is new to you or your family, take it on as a challenge. Ask yourself: What's the most tasty and nutritious treatment I can give to this produce and then teach your kids to do the same.

Kids can learn to be excited about "eating the rainbow" if they discover what each food group does for them. Beneficial plant compounds called *phytonutrients* are typically present in different colored produce. For example:

>> Green fruits and vegetables such as spinach broccoli, kale, green beans, kiwi, Brussels sprouts, and leafy greens promote healthy digestion and heart health while reducing the risk of some cancers.

>> Red fruits and vegetables such as tomatoes, strawberries, cherries, raspberries, and red peppers are believed to reduce the risk of certain cancers while improving vision, strengthening the blood, and promoting heart health.

>> Purple and orange produce such as eggplants, blueberries, blackberries, and purple grapes improve memory and brain function as well as heart health.

>> Orange and yellow produce is believed to improve the immune system and vision while reducing the risk of cardiovascular disease. Carrots, mangoes, sweet potatoes, pineapples, papaya, oranges, and yellow and orange peppers are included in this category.

>> Brown and white plant foods may help in cholesterol management, reducing risk of some cancers and with heart health. These include mushrooms, onions, cauliflower, bananas, parsnips, and others.

TIP

You can help kids to eat the rainbow by basing meals around produce. (It fills them up and gives lots of nutrients as well as in snacks.) While you don't need to give up meat, poultry, or seafood, making sure the produce bases are covered first before filling up the plate with protein alone is best.

The way vegetables are prepared often determines if a child will eat them. We're not saying that you should bread and deep-fry every vegetable so it resembles a fast-food product! Consider these possibilities:

>> Kids often enjoy vegetables that are stir-fried with a little peanut oil or another oil.

>> Vegetables can be pureed into great-tasting soups.

>> Pureed vegetables can also be added to pasta sauce.

>> Most children happily drink vegetable juice.

>> If my granddaughter is any indication, acorn squash can become a kid favorite. (She especially loves it with peas.)

Potatoes are one vegetable that I recommend avoiding because they have a very high glycemic index (see Chapter 16). They are absorbed rapidly and raise your blood glucose rapidly. Also, they are often served fried or with butter and sour cream. So don't push the potatoes.

Cooking Is Cool

There's never been an easier time to get kids interested in cooking than now. With the notion of celebrity chefs on the rise and plenty of cooking shows and reality TV competitions to watch, kids can become very interested in cooking.

Cooking is good for physical and mental health. It's good for physical health because it is a physical activity which can help us burn calories while we do it. Cooking for ourselves also enables us to limit the amount of unhealthy ingredients that go into the food we prepare while boosting the nutrient quotient with good quality ingredients. Our bodies actually crave less food and absorb more nutrients from it when we simply smell foods or hear them being described prior to eating them.

Cooking improves mental health because when we enable it, cooking can provide a daily escape to those actively participating in the task. It doesn't matter if you're only cooking for one, you can still get the benefits of what is now being coined "tasty meditation." *Psychology Today* magazine even cited cooking as a great source of mindful therapy which also provides sensory pleasure.

Teaching kids to cook and to enjoy the kitchen sets them up for a lifetime of creativity, independence, and good nutrition habits.

Tips for getting kids into the kitchen:

>> Adopt a positive attitude for cooking and appreciate the power it has in taking control of our health.

>> Get kids involved in the excitement — share ideas and give them choices from a few different healthy recipes to make.

>> Make it a challenge — how can we make this "insert healthy food name" taste great?

>> Give them tasks: measuring, stirring, rolling, and so on based on age.

>> Let them know how much this means to you and how much you enjoy spending quality time with them — make it a ritual.

Exercise Gives You Energy

Children should be aware of the philosophy "a sound mind in a sound body." You need to inspire your child to actively work on both, and exercise is a great way to do so.

Just like adults, children derive numerous benefits from exercise. Here's a short list you can share with your child:

>> Exercise builds and maintains healthy bones, muscles, and joints.

>> Exercise helps you feel better about yourself.

>> Exercise reduces feelings of stress.

>> Exercise can help you feel more ready to learn in school.

>> Exercise helps you maintain a healthy weight.

>> Exercise helps you sleep better at night.

>> Exercise gives you more energy in general.

Most importantly, know that your child exercises if you do. So get out there and set an example. Remember that every little bit counts, and you don't need an expensive gym membership to exercise. Brisk walking, taking the stairs instead of an elevator, following video exercise programs, and playing sports are all great ways to get more exercise.

Fun Ways to Feel Great

Adopt the mentality that having a positive attitude is good for you and contagious and instill this mentality on your children. Children who maintain a positive attitude simply do better and live a happier life. Teach your child that when they have a positive attitude, they can accomplish whatever they want to do, including being healthy. The ideas in this section work for all ages.

A type of "I spy" game goes a long way into ensuring kids have a positive day, and it starts first thing in the morning. Engage in this activity with your kids by affirming "Today I look for reasons to feel good and I find them," daily. This encourages them (and reminds you) to consistently scan your environment for reasons to be grateful. Teach kids to list and write a gratitude list each morning and/or night.

It's never too early to teach children how to harness the power of happiness hormones to feel better! Dopamine, serotonin, oxytocin, and endorphins are hormones nicknamed the "feel-good hormones" because of the happy and, sometimes, euphoric feelings they create.

Here are a few ways you can help kids to increase production of these hormones:

>> **Dopamine:** The "Reward Chemical" is released when we celebrate small victories, enjoy food, and complete tasks.

>> **Serotonin:** "The Mood Stabilizer" is released with exposure to sun, meditating, running, cycling, and swimming.

>> **Oxytocin:** "The Love Hormone" is released through physical affection such as playing with a baby or dog, holding hands, hugging, expressing and receiving gratitude, and giving compliments.

>> **Endorphins:** "The Pain Killer Hormone" is released through exercise, laughter, aromatherapy, watching a comedy and consuming dark chocolate.

>> **Make it clear to your child that negative thinking is a choice as well.** They can feel bad about a situation, or they can choose to get over it and remind himself that the situation is just temporary.

>> **Helping a child learn a new skill** also increases their self-confidence and self-worth and makes them feel more positive about themself and their world.

>> **Finally, the best way to make your children feel really good about themselves is to constantly remind them with words,** kind gestures, and hugs that they are loved.

Happy Baking Times

Psychologists believe that cooking and baking are therapeutic because they cause behavioral activation, a type of therapy that alleviates depression, anxiety, and attention deficit hyperactivity disorder (ADHD) by increasing goal-oriented behavior and preventing procrastination. The sense of control is mentally empowering, especially for children who otherwise don't have much within their control. When baking bread, kneading and shaping the dough can relieve tension and the process of waiting for the bread to rise can help to promote a sense of delayed gratification.

Chef Amy's happiest childhood memories were spent in the kitchen baking with her Nonna. In her own story, the world of baking became a backdrop for a world of alchemy, tradition, quality time, and loving care that otherwise would have been hard to come by.

Baking, especially bread, is easy and inexpensive. The activity connects us with past and future generations through a technique that is practiced the whole world over. Kids enjoy a great deal of satisfaction when they witness a few staples such as flour, water, yeast, and salt transformed into an edible masterpiece. Plus, by baking items from scratch, you can make sure that you don't have the unhealthful preservatives and additives in them, and feel good about feeding them to your children. See *Diabetes Desserts Cookbook For Dummies* by Amy Riolo for delicious and nutritious ways to enjoy baked goods while balancing your blood sugar.

Playtime with Friends

The foundation of the Mediterranean diet isn't built on food. It's built on eating and enjoying physical activity with others. We should all be doing this daily, so it's never too early to help kids build these skills. Planned playtime with friends and family members can help kids to feel more secure, calm, and connected to others. With everyone's busy schedules nowadays, finding time to socialize is often the lowest on the list of priorities. But with a little effort in the beginning, it can become a healthful trend.

Here are some ways to make sure kids get playtime with friends:

>> Notice pockets in their weeks (especially weekends) when they can socialize

>> Have kids plan to play sports, exercise, or even go on walks with their friends

>> Keep a list of your kids' friends' schedules and discuss play dates with their parents the week prior

>> Start with just one or two playdates a week if necessary and build up to more

If your kids' schedules are already brimming with activities to enjoy with others, pat yourself on the back, you're doing great!

Fresh Air with Family

When we were growing up, fresh air was taken for granted. Kids tended to spend a lot of time outdoors and no special planning was needed to make sure that they got enough exposure to air and sunshine. Nowadays, however, times are different. With all the electronics and technology that kids have at their disposal today, many of them hardly ever go outside. But this is a trend which needs to change.

Mental health experts recommend at least 30 minutes of fresh air per day. Many believe that it's more beneficial to the psyche than antipsychotic drugs. In a world where kids are continuously being diagnosed with social disorders, anxiety, and depression, fresh air offers a lot of benefits including increasing overall health, better mental outlook, improving digestion, immunity, and mood while reducing risk of illness.

The average American spends 90 percent of their life indoors. In the Mediterranean regions where people live longer and healthier, though, people look for any excuse to be outdoors. A British study of 1,000 children found that they were twice as physically active when they were outdoors than indoors. Physical activity, as we discuss earlier in this chapter, is a key factor in reversing and preventing prediabetes.

Light is a mood elevator, and scientists find that just five minutes of exercise in open green spaces resulted in improved mood and self-esteem. Look at your family's schedule and determine times for your kids to be outdoors, even if it is just for a few minutes at a time.

Here are some ideas:

>> Plan meals outdoors when weather permits.

>> Walk around the neighborhood or to do errands as much as possible.

>> Practice outdoor activities — sports, gardening, landscaping, and so on.

>> Spend quality time with kids outdoors — sit on the porch, go to parks, and so forth.

>> Give your indoor spaces as much "outdoor access" as possible — open shades and windows, plant plants and herbs around.

>> Encourage kids to do homework outdoors when weather permits.

Even if you live in a cold or rainy climate, it's worthwhile to bundle up and spend time outdoors. The sun, of course, does offer specific benefits. Sunlight exposure increases our vitamin D, positive emotions, and immunity. It leads to better skin and stronger bones. It also helps us to feel calm and to focus better while preventing or reducing stress, depression, panic attacks, autism, and more.

Researchers at the University of Edinburgh published research which suggests that nitric oxide — a compound naturally produced in skin following sun exposure can help slow weight gain and prevent diabetes. For these reasons, getting kids outdoors again is a great idea!

Index

berberine, 260

bergamot, 261

beta blockers, 90

bioactive compounds, 180, 260, 288

bleached white flour, 59

blood pressure, 77, 81
  diastolic, 89
  levels, 89
  management, 90
  risk, 257
  systolic, 89

blood tests, 259

BMC Endocrine Disorders, 144

body mass index (BMI), 35, 283. *See also* weight gain
  chart, 130
  in children, 96
  familiar with, 128
  level, 29
  and prediabetes, 28
  scores, 129

body weight and shape, prediabetes reversal, 283

bone densitometry study, 145–146

brain health, 18

Brazil nuts, 291

breakfasts recipes
  avocado toast with scrambled eggs, 218, 224–225
  chocolate almond waffles with warm berry compote, 218, 222–223
  citrus yogurt bowl with sweet spices and flax seeds, 217, 220
  cooking, 216–225
  mixed oatmeal and berries with cinnamon and almonds, 217, 219
  savory Mediterranean breakfast platter, 217, 221
  types of, 217

C

calcium, 290

calcium channel blockers, 90

calorie
  definition, 132
  labelling, 57

cancer risk, 19

carbohydrates, 178–179
  absorption of, 257
  diet, 76
  as nutrition, 226, 232
  and prediabetes reversal, 281–282
  refined, 115, 116

cardiovascular diseases risk, 257

cashews, 291

cataracts, 47

catastrophes, 160

Catch-22 (Heller), 149

Centers for Disease Control and Prevention (CDC), 10, 26, 36, 73

Central obesity, 77

CHAOS, 71

cheese, 290

children
  baking interest in, 320–321
  bariatric surgery, 99
  colored plant compounds, 316–317
  cooking interest in, 318

D

E

exercise, 30, 63, 298
  benefits, 143
  to burn glucose, 301–302
  to combat depression, 148–149
  dynamics of, 147
  endorphins level, 149
  equipment, 150
  flexibility, 146
  goal setting, 149
  heart attacks prevention, 144–145
  moderate-intensity, 147
  motivation to, 152
  neurotransmitters level, 148
  osteoporosis prevention, 145–146
  peripheral vascular disease
      prevention, 144–145
  prediabetes reversal, 280
  prediabetes transitioning to diabetes, 144
  resistance, 146
  and sedentary lifestyle, 141–142
  to stop prediabetes, 301–302
  stress, avoidance of, 164
  stroke prevention, 144–145
  three-month plan, weekly plans, 266–274
  tracking, 151–152
  types of, 301–302
  vigorous, 148
  weight-bearing, 146
  weight loss maintenance, 146–148
external locus of control, 162
extra virgin olive oil (EVOO), 286
  in Mediterranean diet, 176–177
eye disease, 46–47
eye health, 17

F

fast food vs real foods, 297
fasting blood glucose
  in children, 97
  definition, 13, 77
  levels of, 14
  normal, 13
  test values, 13
fat, 130, 226, 232
  distribution, 177
  Mediterranean diet, 179–180
  monounsaturated, 117
  in nuts, 292
  polyunsaturated, 117
  and prediabetes reversal, 281–282
  saturated, 117
  subcutaneous, 75
  trans, 117
  treating elevated levels with
      medication, 88
  unsaturated, 117
  visceral, 131
  wrong types of, 117
fertilizers, 111
fiber, 283
  in nuts, 292
  and prediabetes reversal, 281–282
fish
  canned, 289
  fresh, 289
flavonoids, 288
flexibility exercise, 146
follow-up, 37

food
   breakfasts recipes, 216–225
   comfort, 163
   craving, 119, 136, 246, 314
   desserts, 245–251
   fresh, 55–56
   main dishes, 232–245
   and prediabetes reversal, 283
   snacks, 226–231
   stress relationship with, 163
Food and Drug Administration (FDA), 292
food matrix effect, 260
food supply evolution, 110–114
free fatty acids, 75
free radicals, 211
fresh air and nature, 206
Frontiers in Endocrinology, 142
fructose corn syrup, 59, 115
fruits, 283
   in Mediterranean diet, 189
   non-starchy, 287–288

G

gastric banding, 67
gastric bypass, 67
gene expression, 178
genetic predisposition, 74
gestational diabetes, 50, 257
glaucoma, 47
GLP-1 receptor agonists, 52, 64, 257, 258
glucose level
   complications, 33
   control level, 32
   diabetic, 13
   levels of blood, 14, 84

   normal, 13
   prediabetic, 13
   test values, 13
glucose regulation
   exercise and, 147, 301–302
   Mediterranean diet, 175
   prediabetes reversal, 280
   supplements for, 260
glucose tolerance test (GTT), 84
glycemic index (GI), 120, 177–179
glycemic load, 120
glycogen, 147
gratitude, 61, 304
green leafy vegetables, 286–287
gut microbiome, 177

H

Haas, Elson, 92
happiness, 156
hazelnuts, 291
HbA_1C level, 253
   in diabetes diagnosis, 14
   guidelines, 14
   limitations, 84
   prediabetes reversal, 280
   reductions, 258
   reliability, 85
health costs, 21, 22
healthful eating plan, 217
healthy weight
   benefitting from, 125–127
   definition, 127
   diet, 126–127
   exercise, 126–127

heart attacks, 17
  prevention, 144–145
heart disease, 48
Heller, Joseph, 149
herbs, 292–293
  dried, 293
  fresh, 293
high-density lipoprotein (HDL), 86
higher-intensity interval training (HIIT), 30
high fructose corn syrup (HFCS), 59, 115
Hobbs, Christopher, 92
home blood testing kits, 259
hormonal regulation, 178
hormone, 32
hunger, 136
hygiene, 153
hyperosmolar syndrome, 45–46
hypoglycemia
  symptoms, 42
  treatments, 43
  triggers, 42

I

identical twins, 74
impaired fasting glucose (IFG), 14
impaired glucose tolerance (IGT), 14
inflammation, 73, 177
  CRP level, 91
  Mediterranean diet for, 211
  prevention, 226
ingredients list, 58
insulin, 32, 118, 253
  prediabetes reversal and sensitivity, 280
  resistance, 33, 71, 74, 75, 177, 258
    (*see also* metabolic syndrome)
  sensitivity, 33, 177, 260

insurance coverage, 40
interleukin-6 (IL-6), 73
internal locus of control, 162
International Diabetes Federation, 10
It Is So (If You Think So), 161

J

Journal of the American Medical Association (JAMA), 129
joy, 155–157

K

ketoacidosis, 43
  signs, 44
  symptoms, 43–44
  treatment, 44
kidney disease, 47
kidney function, 102

L

labelling, packaged foods, 56
laboratory abnormalities, 78
Lalanne, Jack, 150
legacy effect, 275
lentils, 291
lifestyle changes, 52
  active, 141
  for prediabetes, 28
  progression to diabetes, 279–280
lipoproteins, 86
liraglutide, 52
low-density lipoprotein (LDL), 86
low glycemic index diet, 181

M

macadamia nuts, 291

macronutrients, 217, 226

macrovascular disease, 143–145

magnesium, 259, 290

main dishes, 232–245

management, of prediabetes, 11

management plan, 254

  insulin resistance, 254–255

  lifestyle changes, focus on, 255–256

Managing Cholesterol For Dummies, 81, 175

Mayo Clinic Proceedings, 144–145

meal planning, 266–274, 307–308

meat, 289

medical costs, 21

medications, 40, 52, 64. *See also* supplements

  acarbose, 257

  GLP-1 receptor agonists, 258

  metformin, 256–257

  "off license," 256

  pioglitazone, 257

  recommendations, 256

  side effects, 64, 258

  for treating prediabetes, 284

  weight loss, 258

Mediterranean diet, 137–138, 258, 281, 286, 298–300, 316

  7-day routine planning, 202–209

  ABC's of, 196–197

  affordability, 176

  vs American Diet, 198

  beneficial for prediabetes, 177

  bioactive compounds, 180

  carbohydrates, 178–179

  checklist, 191–195

  as daily routine, 201

  definition, 171–172

  dietary fiber, 186

  environmental benefits, 175

  extra virgin olive oil, 176–177

  fats, 179–180

  fruits and vegetables, 189

  GI Index, 178–179

  for inflammation reduction, 211

  ingredient swap outs for, 197–199

  lexicon, 195–196

  as lifestyle, 190

  lifestyle behind, 184

  plant proteins, 179

  polyphenols, 180

  and prediabetes reversal, 174–175, 180–181, 282

  PREDIMED Mediterranean diet trial, 173

  pyramid, 173, 174

  schedule base template days, 209–210

Mediterranean Lifestyle For Dummies, 185, 191, 204

memory, 101

mental health experts, 36

metabolically obese, 74–75

metabolic syndrome, 29, 32, 71, 73, 74

  causes of, 78–80

  dealing with uncontrolled, 80–81

  definition, 72

  symptoms, 77

metformin, 52, 64, 256–257, 284

Mexican-American ethnicity, 76

microalbumin, 47

microalbuminuria, 78

micronutrients, 259–260

milk, 290

mindful eating, 61

minerals, 259–260, 283

  and prediabetes reversal, 281–282

  source, 93

Mini-Mental State Examination (MMSE), 101

misfortune, 160

monounsaturated fat, 117

Montreal Cognitive Assessment (MoCA), 101

motion disorders, 48

N

napping, 207

National Cholesterol Education Program, 77

National Diabetes Prevention Program (National DPP), 36

National Health and Nutrition Examination Survey (NHANES), 73

National School Lunch Program (NSLP), 123

nerve disease, 48

neurotransmitters level, 148

NHS Diabetes Prevention Program (NHS DPP), 36

nonalcoholic fatty liver disease (NAFLD), 78

nonidentical twins, 74

non-starchy fruits, 287–288

NOVA classification system, 58

nutrition

  benefits, 285

  in children, truth about, 313

  deficiencies, 92

  education on, 313

nuts, 291–292

O

obesity, 65, 77

  in children, 138–139

  visceral, 72

older adults, 283

  diabetes in, 21

  mobility challenges, 30

  prediabetes in, 21

olive oil, 286

  polyphenols, 261

Olive Oil For Dummies, 199, 286

omega-3 fatty acid, 119, 261, 289

omega-6 fatty acid, 119

optic nerve, 47

oral glucose tolerance test (OGTT), 97

origins, of prediabetes, 9

osteoporosis, exercise and prevention of, 145–146

outdoor activities

  children, 321–322

  health and mental wellness, 302–303

overeating, 134

overweight, 129

  and prediabetes, 28

oxidation, 211

oxidative stress, 177, 211

oxytocin, 320

P

packaged foods, 56

peanuts, 291

pecans, 291

peripheral vascular disease, 143

peripheral vascular disease prevention, 144–145

personality traits, 160–161

personal trainers, 36

physical activity, 30, 126–127. *See also* exercise

  7-day routine Mediterranean diet, 206

  in children, 321

  and diseases prevention, 145

  regular, 142

phytonutrients, 316

pioglitazone, 257

Pirandello, Luigi, 161

plant-based/vegetarian diets, 181

plant proteins, 179

plaques, 34

polycystic ovarian syndrome, 17, 78

polyphenols, 226, 288, 292

  in foods, 187–189

  Mediterranean diet, 180

  and prediabetes reversal, 281–282

polyunsaturated fat, 117

Poole, Simon, 204

portion control, 135

positive attitude, 303–304

positive mindset, 211, 264

postmenopausal status, 76

potassium, 290

poultry, 289

prediabetes

  ADA recommendation question, 16–17

  choices, 54

  history of, 15

  mortality, 18

  risks, 17

  tackling through surgery, 65–67

  transition to diabetes, 39

  warning sign for type 2 diabetes, 34

PREDIMED Mediterranean diet trial, 126, 173

pregnancy problems, 50

prevention, progression to diabetes, 279–280, 297–299

probiotics, 261

problem foods to prediabetes connection, 117–120

problem ingredients, 114–117

processed food, 312

  and children, 312–313

  vs real foods, 297

protein, 226, 232

  and prediabetes reversal, 281–282

Q

quality of life, 18

R

Reaven, Gerald, 72

recipes

  almond butter and cinnamon "truffles," 248

  avocado toast with scrambled eggs, 218, 224–225

  blueberry banana smoothie, 227

  breakfast, 216–225

unsaturated fat, 117

US Department of Health and Human Services (HHS), 30

U.S. News & World Report, 172, 183

V

values, test results, 13

vegetables

for children, 313

dietary choices, 316

in Mediterranean diet, 189

very low-density lipoprotein (VLDL), 86

visceral fat, 29, 131

abdominal, 77

vitamins, 259–260, 283

in nuts, 292

and prediabetes reversal, 281–282

quantities, 92

source, 93

supplements, 259–260

vitamin B_{12}, 260

vitamin D, 92, 259

vitamin E, 292

Vitamins For Dummies, 92

W

walking, 63

glucose level and, 302

walnuts, 291

water consumption vs soft drinks, 315

weight gain, 74, 258

management medications, 64

and prediabetes, 28

weight loss

focused diets, 181

maintenance by exercise, 146–148

medications, 258, 284

weight management, 132

World Health Organization (WHO), 57, 77

Y

yogurt, 290

About the Authors

Dr. Simon Poole, MD, has been a primary care physician in Cambridge, England for more than 30 years with a particular interest in public health, lifestyle medicine and nutrition as well as the management of long-term medical conditions. He has taught and undertaken research with Cambridge University and is a founding member of the British and European Associations of Lifestyle Medicine. Simon is a council member of the US True Health Initiative, an International Senior Collaborator with the Global Centre for Nutrition and Health in Cambridge, and was awarded Fellowship of the British Medical Association for services to the profession in 2018, which included longstanding membership of Council of the Royal College of General Practitioners and Public Health Medicine Committee. Simon is a recognized international authority and speaker on lifestyle medicine, chairing the Food Values Conference series at the Pontifical Academy of Science of The Vatican, and the author of the award-winning book *The Olive Oil Diet* (Hachette), *The Real Mediterranean Diet* (Cambridge Academic), *Olive Oil For Dummies, Managing Cholesterol for Dummies,* the latest editions of *Diabetes For Dummies*, *Diabetes Meal Planning & Nutrition For Dummies* and the *Diabetes Cookbook For Dummies* (John Wiley & Sons, Inc.) with Amy Riolo.

Best-selling author **Amy Riolo** is also an award-winning chef, television host, and Mediterranean diet ambassador. The author of 21 books (this is No. 22), she has been named Knight of the Order of the Star of Italy by the Italian government, "The Ambassador of Italian Cuisine in the US" by the Italian International Agency for Foreign Press, "Ambassador of the Italian Mediterranean Diet" by the International Academy of the Italian Mediterranean Diet in her ancestral homeland of Calabria, Italy, and "Ambassador of Mediterranean Cuisine in the World" by the Rome-based media agency *We The Italians*. In 2019, she launched her own private label collection of premium Italian imported culinary ingredients called Amy Riolo Selections and include extra virgin olive oil, balsamic vinegar, and pesto sauce from award-winning artisan companies.

Dedication

Simon Poole: I dedicate my contributions to this book to Sophia Jankula, looking forward to a successful medical career ahead.

Amy Riolo: I dedicate my contributions to this book to my mother, Faith Riolo, for inspiring to learn about diabetes and create diabetes-friendly meal plans and recipes at a young age.

Authors' Acknowledgments

The authors want to thank Tracy Boggier for being so enthusiastic, efficient, and great to work with. We truly appreciate the expert and efficient editorial support and guidance of Thomas Hill and thank Kristie Pyles for all of their support as well. Many thanks to Rachel Nix for her meticulous recipe testing and nutritional analysis.

Dr. Simon Poole: It has been a great honour for me to write another book for the *Dummies* series with Amy, who is a constant source of inspiration and whose alchemy turns medical facts and figures in to practical and delicious recipes for life. I would also like to thank my family and friends who are so supportive in all my endeavours.

Throughout my life, I have been profoundly fortunate to study and work in environments where new evidence is met with curiosity, explored through research, integrated into practice, and, when necessary, questioned with thoughtful critique. This journey began in my childhood in the university town of Aberystwyth, Wales, and continued through my medical studies in London, my clinical practice and public health work in Cambridge, and my engagement with the British Medical Association. I am deeply grateful to the colleagues and mentors, past and present, who embody a commitment to lifelong learning. They have shown me the value of approaching contentious topics with both passion and open-mindedness, and where disagreements arise, responding with patience, courtesy, and compassion. My patients, too, have been among my greatest teachers, imparting invaluable lessons about the importance of respectful listening, shared and informed decision-making, and recognizing individual values and preferences. Their experiences have also reinforced the need to challenge traditional, paternalistic models of medical care. If *Prediabetes For Dummies* offers readers a fresh understanding grounded in these principles, it will be a testament to the many individuals who have shaped my thinking. I remain profoundly indebted to all those who have taught me, and continue to teach me, the enduring importance of curiosity, humility, and empathy in medicine and beyond.

Amy Riolo: My earliest memories of cooking were with my mother, Faith Riolo, who taught me that food was not just something we eat to nourish ourselves, but an edible gift that could be given to express love. When she was later diagnosed with diabetes, it was my love for her and desire to create delicious and nutritious meals for my parents that eventually led me to write books on wellness. I owe much of my professional culinary success to my father, Rick Riolo, for always believing in my talent and supporting my career goals. To my beloved little brother, Jeremy, you are my why, and I'm grateful to be able to pass our family's knowledge down to you.

My nonna, Angela Magnone Foti, taught me to cook and bake, as well as valuable lessons that served me outside of the kitchen. My Yia Yia, Mary Michos Riolo, shared her beloved Greek traditions with me as well. I would probably never have published a cookbook if it weren't for my mentor, Sheilah Kaufman, who patiently taught me much more than I ever planned on learning. I'm proud to pass her knowledge on to others. Without the assistance and guidance of my late friend, spirit sister, and healer Kathleen Ammalee Rogers, I'd never have been able to realize my professional writing goals. I'm very thankful to Chef Luigi Diotaiuti, for always believing in me and for encouraging me to foster my dreams and goals.

There are dozens of people whom I'm proud to call friends and colleagues that I interact with daily and whom each indirectly enable me to achieve my goals. I'm grateful to each of you. I would like to thank Italian President Matarella, Minsistro Gonzalez of the Embassy of Italy in US, and Counselor Michela Carboniero of the Italian Cultural Institute for giving me the honor of being titled Knight of the Order of the Star of Italy." I would also like to thank my dear friends and importers of Amy Riolo Selections products, Stefano and Davide Ferrari for distributing them. Many thanks to all of my wonderful producers; Tenute Cristiano, Olio Anfosso, Pasta Marella, and Acetaia Castelli for their partnerships. In Calabria, Italy I would like to thank my cousins, Angela Riolo, Pina and Franco Riolo, Tonia Riolo, and Mario Riolo for increasing my knowledge and for their support. I would also like to thank Chefs Salvatore Murano and Enzo Murano of Max Trattoria Enoteca for including me in their culinary-cultural pursuits in Italy and for naming me an honorary member of ARCP (Associazione Regionale Cuochi Pittagorici). I am very grateful to the Italian Trade Agency in New York and the Embassy of Italy in Washington, DC for the opportunities and honours that they have bestowed upon me. Mille grazie to Dr. Battista Liserre for his inspirational work on nourishing both the mind and the soul and to Silvestro Parisee for including me in projects which promote Calabria. To my dear friends Jonathan Bardzik, Gail Broeckel, Ann Hotung, Sharon Wolpoff, Jeff Fritz, Ed Donnely, Paul Kolze, Stu Hershey, Maria Fusco, and Kim Foley, you're my spirit family and I'm blessed to have you in my life. Many thanks to Melissa's Produce for their generous donation of produce for recipe development. Many thanks to my tour partner, Alex Safos of Indigo Gazelle Tours for the fantastic opportunities to cook and write in Morocco and Greece. And finally, I would like to thank my co-author, Dr. Simon Poole, for his tremendous knowledge and commitment to the cause of promoting health and happiness, for always inspiring me, and for valuing my voice. It's a pleasure and an honour to collaborate with you.

Publisher's Acknowledgments

Senior Acquisitions Editor: Tracy Boggier

Project Editor: Thomas Hill

Copy Editor: Jerelind Charles

Technical Editor: Dr Gabriele Mocciaro

Recipe Tester and Nutritional Analyst:
Rachel Nix

Production Editor: Bharaneedharan Murthy

Managing Editor: Murari Mukundan

Cover Image: © Sly/stock.adobe.com